SPEECH FACILITATION

SPEECH FACILITATION

Extraoral and Intraoral Stimulation Technique for Improvement of Articulation Skills

By

GWENYTH R. VAUGHN, Ph.D.

Chief, Audiology-Speech Pathology Service
Birmingham Veterans Administration Hospital
Professor, Department of Biocommunication
Schools of Dentistry and Medicine
University of Alabama in Birmingham

and

RUTH MILLBURN CLARK, Ph.D.

Professor Emeritus, University of Denver
Professor Emeritus, Metropolitan State College
Denver, Colorado

CHARLES C THOMAS • PUBLISHER

Springfield • Illinois • U.S.A.

Published and Distributed Throughout the World by

CHARLES C THOMAS • PUBLISHER
Bannerstone House
301-327 East Lawrence Avenue, Springfield, Illinois, U.S.A.

ISBN 0-398-03828-7

Library of Congress Catalog Card Number: 78-16171

Library of Congress Cataloging in Publication Data

Vaughn, Gwenyth R.
Speech facilitation.

Bibliography: p.
Includes index.
1. Articulation disorders. 2. Speech therapy.
3. Phonetics. I. Clark, Ruth Millburn, joint author.
II. Title.
RC424.7.V38 616.8′55′06 78-16171
ISBN 0-398-03828-7

Printed in the United States of America
N-11

CONTRIBUTORS

JOHNNYE AKIN, PH.D.

Professor Emeritus, University of Denver

HERNANDO DE CASTRO, D.D.S., M.S.

Professor, Department of Orthodontics
School of Dentistry
University of Alabama in Birmingham

TED A. FULLER, M.A.

Principal, Speech and Hearing Center
Birmingham Public Schools
Instructor, University College
University of Alabama in Birmingham

ANNE H. B. PUTNAM, PH.D.

Research Associate, Speech Research Laboratory
San Francisco Veterans Administration Hospital

JAMES S. WALL, JR., D.M.D.

General Practice in Dentistry
Huntsville, Alabama

Man's ability to communicate is his most distinctive attribute. It is this capacity which has raised him above all other mammals. From this is derived his capacity to remember the past, to understand the present, and to anticipate the future. It is the core of man's learning and his creative thought.

from—"A Decade of Progress"
NINDB—1961

PREFACE

THE LAST TWO DECADES have witnessed the beginning of extensive research on the peripheral speech mechanism. Some inquiries into the nature of oral sensation and perception have suggested that sensory-perceptual factors may play important roles in the regulation of articulatory functions. As these investigations continue, it is hoped that they will provide the evidence needed to substantiate the long-term clinical success of extraoral manipulations of the speech mechanism in the acquisition, improvement, and maintenance of articulation skills.

Speech clinicians have long sought clinical tools appropriate for assisting persons with articulatory disorders. One of the tools developed was the Moto-kinesthetic Method, a technique utilizing extraoral stimulation. In Speech Facilitation, the extraoral manipulations of the Moto-kinesthetic Method are clarified, additional suggestions are offered, and the preparation and placement of intraoral phonodental guides are described.

Speech Facilitation may be used as a primary or supplementary technique. It is not intended for the refinement of speech but is designed to assist persons with articulatory disorders in the acquisition, improvement, and maintenance of functional articulation skills. The stimulations are prescriptive and may be used in unisensory or in multisensory stimulations.

Speech Facilitation is for use by professional personnel. Supplementary sessions provided by supportive personnel working under close professional supervision may serve as effective reinforcement.

It is recommended that anyone wishing to apply the Speech Facilitation stimulations receive guidance from a clinician experienced in the technique. Before utilizing the stimulations, the stimulator should learn the degree of the pressure, the placement, and the movement appropriate to extraoral manipulations and should become skillful in the placement of phonodental guides. The effectiveness of the stimulations is usually proportional to the skill of the clinician.

SPEECH FACILITATION UTILIZATION

Educational Settings

Speech Facilitation is generally found to be an effective approach to the correction of articulatory defects common to pupils in a public school speech therapy program. Children are easily conditioned to the extraoral manipulations; they learn to initiate the manipulations themselves and to use them as reminders of the position and movement for the target phonemes.

Many clinicians and classroom teachers of preschool and primary school children find Speech Facilitation useful in the programs for developing speech sound awareness.

Most educators of the deaf teach articulation and language skills concomitantly. Those who are familiar with the Speech Facilitation stimulations have found that they usually expedite the learning of the speech sounds for hearing-impaired children and adults.

Speech Facilitation is a valuable tool for assisting mentally retarded persons in the acquisition, improvement, and maintenance of articulatory skills.

Clinical Settings

Speech pathologists familiar with Speech Facilitation find the stimulations helpful in the treatment of persons with severe articulatory disorders related to neurological problems.

Physical, occupational, corrective, educational, and recreational therapists as well as those involved in industrial arts play important roles in supportive activities for persons who have difficulty in acquiring and maintaining functional communication skills. When several members of the health team cooperate in Speech Facilitation programs, their input should be coordinated by speech pathologists trained in the technique.

Home Settings

Coordinated programs utilizing Speech Facilitation may also be arranged with family members and neighbors. During each treatment session, the speech pathologist teaches the manipulations or placement of the guides specific to the target phoneme to the family member accompanying the respondent.

ACKNOWLEDGMENTS

Recognition is given to recent researchers who have diligently studied the sensations and perceptions of the oral cavity and have increased the scientific knowledge and clinical interest in its function as a sensory organ and a motor mechanism.

A debt of gratitude is owed Dr. Edna Hill Young for the development and furtherance of the Moto-kinesthetic Method and to her students who have investigated it and instructed others in its application. Special mention is made of Mrs. Ruth Van Tine who collaborated in the development of a teaching manual and served as a subject in a movie in which Dr. Young demonstrated the Moto-kinesthetic Method.

The authors also wish to thank Anne H. B. Putnam for preparing the first chapter, "Oral Sensations: Basic Review."

The fifth chapter on the preparation and placement of intraoral phonodental guides and use of intraoral cues was prepared with the assistance of Ted A. Fuller, speech pathologist and educator of the deaf, who suggested the design of the stemmed wire guides. The authors also appreciate the assistance of Hernando de Castro, orthodontist, who helped design and who constructed the first sets of stemmed wire guides.

The authors are grateful for the assistance of James S. Wall, Jr., dentist, who designed and placed the first denture guides, and who, in conjunction with Johnnye Akin, professor of phonetics and linguistics, helped in identifying the positions for the dental floss guides. Johnnye Akin also reviewed the phonetic portions of the manual, wrote the introductions to each section in Chapter Six, and suggested "phonodental" as the name for the intraoral guides.

Recognition is given to Hodge Eagleson, physiatrist, who suggested the title Speech Facilitation, to Harry Germagian, medical illustrator, who drew the Manipulation Models, to Craig Luce, medical illustrator, who prepared the diagrams for the phonodental guides, and to Dorothy H. Horton, administrative assistant, who supervised preparation of the manuscript.

G.R.V.
R.M.C.

CONTENTS

TABLE

FIGURES

SPEECH FACILITATION

SECTION I

State of the Art

INTRODUCTION

THE RELATIONSHIPS between physiological events and acoustic products have long posed a challenge to speech scientists; the acquisition, improvement, and maintenance of articulatory skills for persons with communicative disorders have long been of concern to speech pathologists. Careful scrutiny has been given the motor aspects of speech production, but only recently has serious consideration been afforded the effects of sensory inputs upon the articulatory process. Improved treatment programs emerge as scientific fact and clinical findings meld.

Feedback systems reflect changes from within and without. As the senses interact with the environment, they may distort or enhance the messages. Previously, audition and vision were the only senses presumed to play major roles among the sensory systems; touch-pressure, kinesthesis, and proprioception were thought to provide minor input to articulatory functions.

In education, the importance of using the senses was demonstrated by early childhood specialists and by teachers of the deaf and blind. During the last few years, the potential value of touch-pressure, kinesthesis, and proprioception as adjuncts to clinical programs for children and adults with impaired communication skills has begun to be recognized.

Section I Organization

Section I contains three chapters: Chapter 1 gives a basic review of oral sensation. The contribution of oral sensation to motor control of speech is discussed, and a glossary of terms is provided.

Chapter 2 gives a rationale and review of the literature as it relates to sensorimotor, psychodynamic, and learning facilitation.

Chapter 3 includes an historical review of the development and refinement of the Moto-kinesthetic Method and of several intraoral stimulation systems, including intraoral devices.

Chapter 1

ORAL SENSATION: Basic Review

ANNE H. B. PUTNAM

CONTRIBUTION OF ORAL SENSATION TO MOTOR CONTROL OF SPEECH

THE PROCESS OF SPEECH production is a complex sensory-motor phenomenon. In an attempt to construct a working model of the speech production mechanism, speech pathologists and scientists are studying the relative importance of every component in the communication process in order to assign each its appropriate place in the model. This chapter is concerned with the sensory components of the model, and, in particular, the nature and relative contribution of oral sensation to the motor control of speech.

This is not to ignore the importance of auditory sensation to oral communication. The effects of hearing loss, auditory masking, and delayed auditory feedback on the intensity, rate, and resonant quality of speech are notorious. To be sure, appreciation of the contribution of the auditory channel to the speech process has come from many years of observation and experimentation. The importance of the *oral* sensory channel to speech production had, until the last two decades, received less attention than the auditory component. With publication of the Fairbanks model (1954) of the speech production system as a servo mechanism that included feedback from the oral as well as the aural sensors, and subsequent elaborations on that theme (Mysak, 1966; Denes and Pinson, 1966), researchers began to probe the normal range of oral sensory acuity and experimentally alter its parameters. In so doing, a great deal of normative information about the oral sensory mechanism was compiled for use in assessing the oral sensory skills of talkers with pathological oral communication skills.

The speech pathologist has been bombarded with exhortations to consider articulation problems in light of possible oral sensory deficits, to test oral sensory abilities in their clients, and to drill for improvement of oral sensory skills. Language clinicians have been warned not to exclude the oral sensory channel when developing sensory/motor skills in language impaired children. Unfortunately, in many cases, adequate definitions of the oral sensory modalities that are accessible to testing and modification have been overlooked, and the issue has been confused by ambiguous or inaccurate terminology. The intent of the material that follows is to describe as clearly as possible those oral sensations that relate to oral motor skill and to delineate what is known about the level of their influence in the central nervous system.

Definition of Terms

The general senses of the oral and perioral tissues include pain, temperature, touch-pressure, kinesthesis, and proprioception. The last three of these are pertinent to this discussion, and at the outset, the terms must be clarified. (It is recognized that there are exceptions to the generalizations made in the task of definition. The definitions offered here are those most commonly used by contemporary investigators.)

TOUCH-PRESSURE. The sensation of *touch-pressure* (including light touch, deep pressure, taction, and vibrotaction), is a sensitivity to the mechanical contact of objects with the surface of the body. Touch-pressure is received *via* mechanoreceptors in the skin, fascia, and deep tissues, exclusive of the muscles and joints (Mountcastle and Darian-Smith, 1968). By virtue of touch-pressure sensitivity, one can judge the intensity, location, contour and/or temporal rhythm of a mechanical stimulus.

KINESTHESIS. Kinesthesis is the sensation of rate and direction of body-part movement as well as discrimination of steady position and is thought to be monitored by mechanoreceptors in and about the joint capsules and ligaments (Mountcastle, 1968). Kinesthetic sensations are integrated with information from the visual and vestibular systems for the concept of total body-form and position in space. Conscious touch-pressure and kinesthetic sensations together constitute *somesthetic* sensations which must be integrated in sensory tasks such as stereognosis (form discrimination).

PROPRIOCEPTION. Proprioception, which consists of neural information on the length and tension of muscles, is generally thought to be monitored by muscle spindles and tendon organs (Henneman, 1968). A major organizational component of proprioception is the gamma loop that circuits between muscle spindles and brain stem and/or cerebellum, and back again to the muscles. Proprioceptive sensory fibers constitute the afferent part of the loop; gamma motor fibers complete the efferent part of the loop. This system aids in the reflexive control of initial acceleration of movement, overshoot, and tension regulation in skeletal muscles (for a detailed discussion of muscle spindles and gamma loops, see Matthews, 1964; Bowman, 1971; Abbs, 1973).

Feedback

According to Hardy (1970), feedback from the senses cited above communicates with the central nervous system at three levels during speech production. A certain amount of *reflexive* oral motor activity is thought to depend on proprioception conveyed from muscle spindles and tendon organs to the cervical spinal cord and brain stem. The much-talked-about gamma loop is probably a major functor at this unconscious reflex level. At a more complex, but still unconscious level of servocontrol, the thalamus and cerebellum monitor afferent impulses for the coordination of efferent neuromotor activity. Tactile (hereafter synonymous with *unconscious* touch-pressure sensation) and proprioceptive information are thought to be prime sensory contributors to speech motor control at these subcortical levels. At the level of the cortex, in the region of the post-central gyrus, afferent impulses relaying touch-pressure (hereafter synonymous with *conscious* touch-pressure sensation) and kinesthesis from the articulators contribute to the conscious perception of oral somesthesis and its discriminable dimensions. It must be pointed out, however, that within the peripheral speech production apparatus, the physiological distinctions among these various sensations and the organs that subserve them are neither clear-cut nor completely understood.

MECHANORECEPTORS. It is well established that the oral structures, particularly the lips and the tongue, are richly endowed with mechanoreceptors innervated by the trigeminal and/or glossopharyngeal nerves. Hence, the touch-pressure and tactile sensitivity of these tissues has been found to be extremely keen. Touch-pressure acuity is highest in the front of the mouth, particularly on the tongue tip and lips, and decreases as the stimulus moves posteriorly in the oral cavity. The touch-pressure sensitivity in any given oral tissue is directly related to the density of mechanoreceptors in the tissue and to the size of the areas in the thalamus and sensory cortex devoted to oral sensory perception from that region (Grossman, Hattis, and Ringel, 1965).

Oral kinesthesis is also keen but is a more complicated issue than touch-pressure. A primary source of kinesthesis in the supraglottic region is the temporo-mandibular joint which conveys mandibular position information *via* the trigeminal nerve. The intrinsic lip and lingual muscles, however, have no jointed skeletal elements by which to convey movement and position sensations. It has been suggested that muscle spindles may contribute to kinesthesis from these tissues, but this is a moot point in view of the fact that muscle spindles are not thought to contribute to conscious sensation and perception. A more reasonable suggestion is that conscious awareness of tongue and lip movements and positions is a function of cutaneous and deep mechanoreceptors (Cooper, 1953; Bowman, 1971; Leanderson, 1972). According to Sybil Cooper (1953), touch-pressure receptors may provide information to the cortex that is "used in a similar way to kinesthetic information from joints and periosteal endings" (p. 198). This is a valid suggestion in view of the fact that a trigeminal nerve block not only substantially reduces touch-pressure sensitivity in the anterior oral structures but also blocks the subjective perception of tongue and lip position, rates, and directions of movement (Scott and Ringel, 1971; Putnam and Ringel, 1976).

MUSCLE SPINDLES. The least well understood aspect of oral sensation is proprioception. The only point on which most experimenters agree is that such afferent information on the length and tension of muscles is utilized only at subcortical levels; hence, proprioceptive acuity, *per se,* is difficult to assess because it functions at a subconscious level to coordinate motor activity. The muscles of mastication have good spindle endowments, and James H. Abbs (1973) has been able to demonstrate experimentally that proprioception from mandibular muscle spindles is used to regulate the initiation, velocity, and temporal control of jaw movements during speech.

With respect to the tongue and lips, the contribution of muscle spindles to proprioception for motor control is less clear-cut. The existence of spindle organs in the tongue has long been a controversial issue, primarily because spindles are not distributed uniformly throughout the lingual musculature and hence are not readily seen in every histological section. They are generally recognized to exist in substantial numbers in the extrinsic tongue musculature. Furthermore, the histological data of Cooper (1953) suggest that spindles are numerous in the superior longitudinal, transverse, and vertical intrinsic muscle fibers of the tongue immediately behind the tip, along the dorsal mid-line, and near the lateral margins. Spindles are scarce, apparently, in the inferior longitudinal muscles and in the tongue's tip and back tissue. The path of afferent fibers from lingual muscle spindles has also created controversy. Some evidence (Hosokawa, 1961; Konigsmark, 1970) suggests that the spindle afferents leave the tongue *via* the hypoglossal nerve trunk (Cranial Nerve XII). This cranial nerve has no sensory root, however, and any afferent fibers that it might carry are thought to enter the central system *via* the dorsal roots of the first few cervical nerves. Other investigators have argued that spindle afferents leave the tongue *via* the lingual branch of the trigeminal nerve (Cranial Nerve V).

Proprioception in the facial muscles, including the lips, is also an ambiguous issue. The existence of functional spindle organs in these muscles is questionable (Hosokawa, 1961; Leanderson, 1972). In the absence of true proprioceptors in the form of spindle organs, the lips are thought to rely on mechanoreceptors for proprioception as well as somesthesia. It is known that somesthesia and tactile sensations in facial tissues are subserved by the trigeminal nerve, but the path of afferents from intradermal or subcutaneous "proprioceptors" is not clearly understood. It is possible that they proceed to the brainstem *via* the facial nerve (Hosokawa, 1961) and hence would not be affected by a trigeminal injury or experimental nerve block, but this remains unresolved (Baumel, 1974).

The foregoing information on lingual and labial sensory function is summarized in Table I.

Oral Sensory Deprivation

Bosma's symposia (1967, 1970, 1972) on oral sensation and perception have included reports on talkers with congenital sensory deficits involving the oral tissues (Chase, 1967; Rootes and MacNeilage, 1967; Zlatin, 1972). Such cases are rare, however, and generalizations made from them as to the importance of adequate oral sensation and per-

TABLE I*

SUMMARY OF PROPRIOCEPTIVE, TACTILE, AND SOMESTHETIC SENSORY FUNCTIONS IN THE LIPS AND ANTERIOR TWO THIRDS OF THE TONGUE

Sense	*Receptor Organ*	*Peripheral Pathway*	*Central Connections*
Proprioception	Muscle spindles Tendon organs	Tongue: hypoglossal or trigeminal nerve	Cervical cord, or brain stem and cerebellum
		Lips: facial or trigeminal nerve	Brain stem and cerebellum
Taction	Cutaneous and deep tissue mechanoreceptors	Trigeminal nerve	Brain stem and cerebellum
Kinesthesis	Cutaneous and deep tissue mechanoreceptors	Trigeminal nerve	Lemniscal system, thalamus, and postcentral gyrus of cortex
Touch-pressure	Cutaneous and deep tissue mechanoreceptors	Trigeminal nerve	Lemniscal system, thalamus, and postcentral gyrus of cortex

* Compiled from information presented by Cooper, 1953; Mountcastle and Darian-Smith, 1968; Henneman, 1968; Mountcastle, 1968; Hardy, 1970; and Leanderson and Persson, 1972.

ception to speech development are imprudent since such congenital sensory neuropathies are often complicated by other unknown neurological and/or developmental aberrations.

In the laboratory, in an effort to assess the effect of oral sensation loss on oral motor performance, researchers have induced oral sensory deprivation temporarily by means of nerve block injections (McCroskey, 1958; Ringel and Steer, 1963; Gammon, Smith, Daniloff and Kim, 1971; Scott and Ringel, 1971; Abbs, 1973; Borden, Harris and Catena, 1973; Hutchinson and Putnam, 1974; Putnam and Ringel, 1976). The nerve most often used for such research in humans is the trigeminal. In light of the preceding discussion about oral sensations, however, and recent research (Abbs, Folkins, and Sivarajan, 1976), it is apparent that the effects of an experimental trigeminal nerve block on oral sensation and perception will be somewhat ambiguous. The mandibular, lingual, infraorbital, and palatine nerve injections which constitute the typical experimental trigeminal block are thought to reduce substantially the sensitivity of mechanoreceptors in the lips, teeth, alveolar ridges, palates, oral mucosa, and anterior two-thirds of the tongue. In terms of sensory modalities, such a block abolishes touch-pressure and taction in those tissues. And, insofar as mechanoreceptors in the tongue and lips may monitor kinesthesis, the probability exists that it is blocked as well. It is not known how much, if any, proprioception is blocked by the anesthesia. Presumably, subjects are left with access to a certain amount of oral sensory feedback in the form of (1) proprioceptive information from muscle spindles in the muscles of mastication, *via* an unblocked portion of the trigeminal nerve; (2) kinesthetic information from the temporo-mandibular joint, *via* an unblocked portion of the trigeminal; (3) the possibility of proprioceptive information from extrinsic and intrinsic tongue muscle spindles, assuming that they are innervated by the hypoglossal nerve; and (4) proprioception from intradermal mechanoreceptors in the labial and facial musculature, assuming these are innervated by the facial nerve (Putnam and Ringel, 1973).

Testing Oral Sensation

In the process of our attempts to understand more about oral sensation and perception, a number of methods have evolved by which to assess conscious oral sensory abilities; that is, touch-pressure and kinesthesis. (Proprioception in the strict sense of the word is the sensation from muscle spindles and tendon organs that functions to regulate motor activity at subconscious and reflexive levels; hence it is not readily available for assessment in the conscious patient. The word "proprioception" is also often used, however, in the general sense to describe a conscious awareness of body-part position in space and movement.) Threshold tests do exist for the sensation of light pressure, light touch, and vibrotaction. Discrimination tests are available for two point contacts, weight, mandibular kinesthesis (openness of jaw), lingual kinesthesis (tongue tracking and pattern recognition paths), and textures. In addition, tests of oral stereognostic abilities are available. These are form recognition or discrimination tasks performed in the mouth and require the integration of oral touch-pressure and kinesthetic sensation (see Ringel, 1970; Williams and LaPointe, 1971 a and b).

Oral Stereognosis

Tests of oral stereognosis have attracted particular attention in the last several years when it was found that in some talkers, poor oral stereognostic performance accompanied persistent speech articulation problems for which there was no organic explanation. That is, some clients who had been in articulation therapy for months without improvement demonstrated poor oral stereognostic abilities on oral form tests. Further, the work of Robert Ringel and his colleagues (Ringel, Burk, and Scott, 1968; Ringel, 1970) demonstrated that oral form testing could distinguish among talkers with articulatory defects in terms of the severity of the articulation problems and kinds of oral stereognostic discrimination errors they made. These persons with articulatory defects and poor oral stereognostic abilities, however, did not necessarily demonstrate a deficit in either touch-pressure or kinesthetic acuity when these modalities were tested separately. While the neurophysiological relationship between oral form discrimination ability and articulation proficiency is not thoroughly understood, it has been hypothesized that in cases of talkers who are poor in both regards, the astereognosis may not result from a particular sensory deficit, *per se*, but rather from a subtle disorder in the client's ability to integrate the touch-pressure and kinesthetic feedback needed for adequate performance on oral stereognostic tests; the same subtle disorder may be responsible, to some degree, for the articulation problem when the client's inability to integrate the somesthetic cues that produce an acute awareness of spatial and temporal relationships among the oral structures renders his fine motor control for speech less than adequate for some difficult articulatory maneuvers.

In a few cases, oral stereognostic training has actually been incorporated into articulation therapy with good results, and as a client's oral form discrimination abilities have improved, so has the heretofore resistant articulation defect. Using oral stereognostic training as an adjunct to articulation therapy for some subjects appears to provide a means to an end, but not an end in and of itself; and it has not been successful in all cases. When it has been used with success, it has appeared to improve a subject's awareness of spatiotemporal structural relationships within the oral cavity and to facilitate his ability to handle touch-pressure and kinesthetic sensations from the oral structures. It is reasonable to hypothesize that such heightened awareness and improved skill may be generalized to speech tasks as well.

NEED FOR RESEARCH

For over a quarter of a century, Edna Hill Young demonstrated the need to utilize oral sensation in the treatment of articulation disorders. In the decades of the 1950s and 1960s, Ruth Clark and her students explored and reported the literature related to oral sensation and speech. About the same time, speech scientists began to explore the oral sensory channels experimentally.

While much is now known theoretically about the oral sensations, an understanding of the accessibility and utility of these sensations in the oral and perioral tissues for the development and maintenance of articulatory skills is far from complete. There is enough scientific information, however, to say that the oral sensory channels should *not* be neglected or overlooked in speech habilitation or rehabilitation.

Continued research efforts in clinics and laboratories into the relative contributions of oral sensations to speech and their utility in the face of auditory, visual and/or oral deficits will, hopefully, shed more light on the understanding of the unique oral sensory attributes of the speech production mechanism.

GLOSSARY OF TERMS

HAPTIC PROCESSING: Haptic processing is the processing of touch-pressure sensations.

KINESTHESIS: Kinesthesis is the general somatic sensation of the rate and direction of body-part movement as well as the ability to discriminate steady position. It is monitored *via* mechanoreceptors in the joint capsules and ligaments.

MECHANORECEPTORS: Mechanoreceptors are sensory receptors that respond to mechanical force, e.g., pressure, vibration, or stretch. They take essentially three forms: specialized non-neural cells (encapsulated endings); organized nerve endings (expanded tips); or free peripheral endings of afferent nerve fibers.

Mechanoreceptors serve as *touch-pressure* sensors *via* organized and free nerve endings in the skin, fascia, periosteum, and tendon capsules, e.g., Merkel's discs, Ruffini's endings, Meissner's corpuscles, Krause's end bulbs, pacinian corpuscles, and Golgi-Mazzoni endings.

Mechanoreceptors serve as *kinesthetic* sensors in the joint capsules and ligaments *via* organized nerve endings of the Golgi or Ruffini type.

Mechanoreceptors serve as *proprioceptive* sensors in muscles (spindle organs) and tendons (Golgi tendon organs).

Mechanoreceptors are also found in the cochlear and vestibular organs of the inner ear and serve as visceral pressure receptors in portions of the circulatory system.

MUSCLE SPINDLES AND TENDON ORGANS: Muscle spindles and tendon organs are highly specialized mechanoreceptors located in the fleshy belly of the muscle and the musculotendinous junctions, respectively.

The spindles, oriented "in parallel" with the muscle fibers, and the tendon organs, oriented "in series" with the muscle fibers, together provide subconscious levels of the central nervous system with proprioceptive feedback on the length, tension, and velocity of stretch in muscles. Muscle spindles are also essential components of the gamma motor system's servo control of the initial acceleration of movement, overshoot, and tension regulation in skeletal muscle.

ORAL STEREOGNOSIS: Oral stereognosis provides perception of the size and shape of three-dimensional objects placed in the mouth for exploration. The task of oral stereognosis depends on the integration of touch-pressure and kinesthetic sensations from the perioral and intraoral tissues used in exploration of the object. This perceptual ability can be tested in a recognition paradigm where the subject matches the perceived spatial characteristics of a form explored in the mouth with an array of similar sizes and shapes perceived visually (intersensory matching task). Stereognosis can also be tested in a discrimination paradigm in which objects are presented for intraoral exploration in pairs, and same/different judgements are made by the subject based only on his oral sensory perceptions about the size and shape of one object compared to the other (intrasensory discrimination task).

PROPRIOCEPTION: Proprioception consists of subconscious sensory information on the length and tension of muscles and the velocity of stretch. It is provided by mechanoreceptors in the muscles and tendons that are sensitive to stretch. Proprioception constitutes the afferent portion of the gamma loop which functions in the reflexive control of tension regulation and motion refinement in skeletal muscles.

TOUCH-PRESSURE (touch, taction, light pressure): Touch-pressure is the general somatic sensation of mechanical deformation of the surface of the body. It is received *via* mechanoreceptors in the cutaneous tissues and in some deep tissues exclusive of muscles and joints. The quality of touch-pressure sensations can be quantified along several different perceptual parameters including place, intensity, contour, and temporal pattern of the mechanical stimulus.

Chapter 2

RATIONALE AND REVIEW OF THE LITERATURE

- SENSORIMOTOR FACILITATION
  - Touch-Pressure
  - Kinesthesis
  - Haptic Processing
  - Proprioception
  - Audition
  - Vision
  - Sensorimotor Isomorphism
  - Speech and Sensorimotor Defects
- PSYCHODYNAMIC FACILITATION
  - Body Percept
  - Self Concept and Speech
    - Stutterers
    - Laryngectomees
- LEARNING FACILITATION
  - Learning Theory
  - Behavior Modification
- Summary Statement

SENSORIMOTOR FACILITATION

SINCE THE MIDDLE FIFTIES, threads of information concerning the impact of touch-pressure, kinesthesis, and proprioception upon the articulation of speech sounds appear in the literature. Hopefully, these strands will ultimately form a fabric that will be strong enough to sustain scientific scrutiny as well as clinical application. When this occurs, clinicians will be better able to guide their clients in the acquisition, improvement, and maintenance of articulation skills.

The following is a review of studies concerned with the roles of tactile, kinesthetic, proprioceptive, auditory, and visual processes, and their probable contribution to the enhancement or deterioration of the ultimate articulatory product.

Touch-Pressure

Gerald McCall (1969) postulated that there were at least four tactile skills that appeared to have relevance to the acts of speaking, chewing, and swallowing: (1) detection of the presence of tactile stimuli and appreciation of minimal changes in tactile stimulation, (2) spatial discrimination and localization of tactile stimuli, (3) temporal discrimination of tactile stimuli, and (4) appreciation of simultaneous bilateral tactile stimuli.

James F. Bosma, in *Symposium on Oral Sensation and Perception* (1967), stressed that sensitivity of the tongue tip to tactile and two-point discrimination was greater than in any other body area, even that of the fingertips. Bosma felt that, in spite of the enormous volume of tactile experience, the mouth continued to perform as a single sensorimotor organ, effecting a unity of function. He indicated, however, that the highest level of sensorimotor integration in the oral area had, till then, defied analysis.

In 1970, Bosma, in the *Second Symposium on Oral Sensation and Perception,* stated that human and other mammalian neonates accomplished their most skilled environmental manipulation and best demonstrated their capacity for learning at their mouths.

In the second Bosma volume (1970), research concerning oral activity that had been carried on during the prenatal period was reported. The study by Tryphena Humphrey on reflex activity of the oral and facial areas of the human fetus included film studies of 159 human fetuses and showed that "total pattern reflexes" were elicitable from the maxillary and mandibular nerves at 7.5 weeks and became progressively more discriminate and more varied in the period leading up to suckling (twenty-four weeks). Humphrey and others stated in the *Symposium* that touch developed earlier and matured long before the ears, eyes, and higher brain centers. The investigators indicated that prenatally, as well as postnatally, the mouth tended to open when the lips were touched and that other mouth opening reflexes, especially those that included tongue movements and swallowing, became a part of the complex reactions that later developed into feeding and respiratory activities.

Humphrey believed that the central nervous system as well as the peripheral receptors were important in the perception of any sensation. Although the reactions of the systems differed in complexity, many of the sequences in which fetal movements developed were repeated postnatally.

In the *Third Symposium on Oral Sensation and Perception,* edited by Bosma in 1972, a number of papers were included that focused entirely on the mouth of the infant. These papers treated the mouth and pharynx as one organic unit and emphasized that they must work very well together or malfunction would take place. It was pointed out, however, that when structures were defective, the organism had a remarkable capacity for compensation.

Joan Wilentz (1968) wrote that touch was extremely important to the young baby in feeding, investigating, and reacting to his environment. She pointed out that the tactual sense was so crucial that it might be said that in the first years of life, man was educated by touch.

James A. Carrell (1968) stated that:

> To learn articulation, the infant must have normal sensitivity to auditory, kinesthetic, and tactile stimuli. He must first of all hear speech in his environment in order to learn to talk, and the self-stimulation provided by babbling and vocal play is vital in establishing the feedback loops. As he plays with the sounds of speech and later, when he learns to combine them into words, other sensory modalities become important. He unconsciously learns to feel the articulation movements through kinesthesia and through the tactile stimuli of the tongue, lip, and palate surfaces in contact with each other and stimulated by breath flow. These afferent stimuli, integrated at higher levels, thus become incorporated into the feedback loops (p. 9).

Kinesthesis

As early as 1942, Frances Patton wrote about the importance of the kinesthetic sense in speech acquisition. She stated that this sense was of basic importance in learning speech and that without it the conditioned reflex of speech would probably not be established or maintained. Patton felt that the kinesthetic sense gave a person an awareness of position and tenseness of the organs involved in speech production and that these impressions helped arouse motor impulses for speech which were, in turn, evaluated by the auditory sense. Patton also said that before a sound or group of sounds could be produced at will, sufficient repetition was needed to create a kinesthetic memory. Patton stated that the kinesthetic sense was basically important in the first stages of speech.

Eugene McDonald and Lester Aungst (1967) indicated that a speech pathologist needed to understand (1) the nature of speech movements, (2) how these movements were activated and controlled, and (3) the sequences in which the speech producing movements were learned.

Haptic Processing

The integration of cutaneous and kinesthetic information is sometimes referred to as "haptic perception." When external stimuli, whether imposed on a passive subject or self-initiated, comes in contact with the skin, and when muscular or skeletal movement occurs, the haptic system is activated. Upon either active or passive stimulation, the sense organ's "mechanoreceptors" are activated.

In a review of research on *Central Processing Dysfunction in Children,* James C. Chalfant and Margaret A. Scheffelin (1969) discussed haptic processing. They stated that a great deal of information is available concerning auditory and visual input channels, but "there is comparatively little information concerning the processing of cutaneous (touch) and kinesthetic (body movement) information." They deplored this situation since touch and body movement have proved to be very useful in teaching deaf, blind, and deaf-blind children. They felt there was a need "to investigate the potential value of touch and movement for teaching children who can hear and see" (p. 39).

Chalfant and Scheffelin (1969) described "haptic processing" as the integration of cutaneous kinesthetic information and "haptic perception" as the result of central processing of the synthesis of cutaneous and kinesthetic information.

In 1967, Gibson stated that the simultaneous input of cutaneous and kinesthetic perception provided more informational input than either system alone, including "(1) dynamic movement patterns of the trunk, arms, legs, mandible, and tongue; (b) static limb positions or postures; and (c) sensitivity to the direction of linear and rotary movement of the skull, limbs, and entire body" (pp. 111-136).

Proprioception

Joan S. Wilentz (1968), exploring the many senses in man, said that the impulses were triggered by proprioceptions. She stated that these impulses were carried by some of the fastest conducting nerves in the body and achieved velocities of between 200 and 300 feet per second.

James Tyson (1954) suggested the somesthetic pathways to the parietal lobes were employed by sensations resulting from touch, pressure, and movement stimulation of the exteroceptors and muscle-stretch and muscle-contraction stimulation of the proprioceptors. He felt that through (1) the initiation of the muscle movements related to the production of normal speech sounds, and (2) the synchronization of these movements with auditory and visual stimulation, the most complete mnemonic neural patterns possible were produced. According to Tyson, the parietal lobe, with its associated somesthetic sensations, appeared to be an excellent projection area for the integration of sensations with motor response. He described the auditory, the visual, and the somesthetic cortex as constituting a triumvirate of sensory mediators that lay down, in conjunction with the motor cortex, useful neural patterns for desired future muscle movement.

Helen Dittman (1955) studied the importance of proprioceptive sense to speech production. She concluded that because of its automatic nature, little consideration was given to proprioceptive control when the central nervous system was normal. She postulated that this sense was often neglected in the training program of those who did not have normal speech because of the lack of recognition and the apparent subservient status of proprioception to the other senses.

A number of investigators have suggested that speech is initially built upon proprioceptive sensations that come from reflexive activities such as sucking, swallowing, vomiting, yawning, and others. Dittman (1955) indicated that the physical climate for the facilitation of normal reflexive action and the future support for vocal activity was dependent on the stimulation of the various proprioceptive sensibilities of pressure, stretch, movement, and on control of mass reflexes. She concluded that proprioception was fundamental to speech at any stage of development. She believed that an individual became aware of muscle tension and a positional sense as he received, during speech activity, a continuous series of proprioceptive impressions at either the conscious or unconscious level and that these impressions helped arouse motor impulses to guide the speech organs through the related acts of speaking. According to Dittman, speech, although complicated by the ideational and emotional aspects of language, was basically a motor activity for which the proprioceptive sense, in conjunction with the auditory, tactual, and visual senses, was fundamental. She said that the sensations appeared to be of such an automatic nature in normal speech production that they were unrecognized and usually were not emphasized in the rehabilitation process. She felt that all speech involved muscle activity and all muscle activity involved proprioception.

Mildred Berry (1969) described the primary importance of proprioception and said that it employed bi-directional tracts in the nervous system that might more properly be called sensorimotor loops.

The concept of moto-kinesthetic feedback loops as essential to the comprehension and use of language was recognized by Alvin M. Liberman (1957).

Some specialists in physical medicine and rehabilitation proposed that proprioceptive sensibilities be stimulated in adults to augment the habilitation and rehabilitation of persons suffering from neuromuscular disorders. Hodge Eagleson (1972) suggested that the actual movements in the performance of an act itself might be the preferred type of exercise.

Audition

For years, audition was considered the chief modality in the perception of speech. Grant Fairbanks (1954) postulated the importance of kinesthetic, auditory, and tactile feedback in a speech servomechanism. He hypothesized that proper speech production required information from the kinesthetic sensory system. Charles Van Riper and John Irvin (1958) and Edward Mysak (1959) concurred with Fairbanks. These authors pointed out that improper functioning of the input channels might result in disordered speech output. Van Riper and Irvin theorized that the tactile or kinesthetic feedback channels probably replaced the auditory channel as the main monitoring agent after speech developed and that, thereafter, feedback through the ear, though still active, assumed a secondary role.

Numerous investigators studied the importance of the tactile system (Shelton, Arndt, and Hetherington, 1967; Arndt, Gauer, Shelton, Crary, and Chisum, 1970; Williams and LaPointe, 1971 a and b; Locke, 1968; Liberman, 1957; and Morley and Fox, 1969). Several suggested that the tactile and kinesthetic monitoring systems were more vital in the perception of articulatory placement than audition, once speech patterns had been established (McDonald, 1967; McCall, 1969; and Carrell, 1968). The motor theory of speech perception (Liberman, 1957) maintained that articulatory movements and their sensory feedback mediated between the acoustic stimulus and the perception of speech.

Research reviewed by Berry (1969), however, indicated that a child perceived sound sequences in terms of his own motor reactions. Berry stressed that this statement did not imply that acoustic events were unimportant, but that they were linked in time with the equally important articulatory events.

Hardy (1970) commented that auditory monitoring was of importance to the development of and maintenance of speech production.

He pointed out that deaf children routinely did not develop speech production capability.

Many investigators contended that the auditory signal was a component of the total sensory experience associated with speech generation and that it contained important information related to the "target" or end product of speech musculature patterning. Thus, they reasoned, most congenitally deaf and adventitiously deafened persons had difficulty in learning and maintaining many of the components of the speech signal respectively. The deterioration of speech in the latter group usually occurred in those speech elements requiring the most precise muscular patterning, such as the consonants. Vowels were usually not affected until later (Carhart, 1960).

Since the blocking of auditory feedback process by masking routinely showed little disruption of articulatory capability, it was concluded that intraoral sensations could provide cues for positioning of the speech musculature once the appropriate patterning had been learned, and that they could continue to do so in the absence of auditory feedback (Hardy, 1970).

Vision

Gibson (1967) stated that visual input dominated the haptic system in awareness. He also said that skin-joint sensitivity was inevitable and that the latter made an even more fundamental contribution to the control of motor skill than vision.

He described the mouth as an active perceptual system that included a set with overlapping parts consisting of lips, jaw, teeth, tongue, palate, and throat, all having a complex musculature.

He referred to the mouth as a complex organ system for vocalizing that later developed the capacity for speaking.

In 1940, Thomas Ryan wrote about the interrelationships of the sensory systems in perception. He said that while one modality usually predominated, most objects were perceived through two or more sensory modalities working in cooperation. He also stated that sensory systems were by no means insulated from one another but were parts of a unified organism. Ryan gave the example of a person seeing an iron object and perceiving it to be heavy. The visual perception was thus integrated with the tactual as a part of a total situation. Ryan also indicated that outside of the controlled conditions of a laboratory, it was extremely rare for even a single object to be the product of the operation of a single sensory system.

Sensorimotor Isomorphism

Charles F. Osgood (1968) described the general principle of isomorphism in which anatomical projections of the various body parts in the sensory and motor cortices of the brain were correlated in juxtaposition and with functional interconnection. Further, Osgood postulated that feedback or conditioning relationships existed between stimuli or sensory signals and between responses or motor signals. He proposed the psychological theory that patterning, regularities, and ordering of events in the stimulating environment of an organism were mirrored in its sensory nervous system.

Bosma (1970) stated that human speech was the greatest achievement in intermodal afferent guidance of oral actions. He also pointed out that the brain had known the mouth in all stages of development, that oral function was affected by this relationship, and that the anatomical mouth was modulated in dimension and proportioned reciprocally so that the cerebrum's discriminations of functions were effected.

Speech and Sensorimotor Defects

A comparative study by Mark Larson (1955) focused upon the kinesthetic and tactile abilities of normally speaking subjects and subjects having "functional" articulation problems. He suggested that a poor "feel" for speech resulted in some "functional" articulation problems. He found that the normally speaking control group's superiority over the group with "functional" articulation problems was decidedly significant. He concluded that the tactile aspects of speech production might be useful in therapeutic procedures.

Robert Ringel and Stanley Ewanowski (1965) suggested a relationship of disturbed oral tactile perception to the high incidence of lingual agnosia in speech defectives.

According to McDonald and Aungst (1967), preliminary research findings and clinical observations encouraged the speculation that there might well be a subgroup of persons with defective oral motor function such as poor articulation or poorly developed chewing, sucking, and swallowing, whose motor dysfunction might be associated with defective oral sensory abilities.

Bosma (1967) explored the role of oral sensation and perception in the control of oral activities. He identified the need for increased understanding of complex sensorimotor actions of the mouth. He mentioned the apparent correlation between oral stereognosis and speech articulation but warned that research was needed to clarify the mechanism of central integration and its relationship to oral stereognosis and articulation. Additional research is listed in *References* (Class, 1956; Press, 1975).

PSYCHODYNAMIC FACILITATION

Body Percept

Paul Schilder (1950) pointed out the importance of body percept and "body image" related to normal and abnormal behavioral function. Seymour Wapner and Heinz Werner edited a volume that grew out of a symposium, *The Body Percept,* in 1965. The authors discussed problems related to body experience. A variety of terms were used by the different participants such as, "body percept," "body concept," and "body image." Such broad psychological functions as abstract thought, perception, emotion, personality, body image boundary, symbolization, and motor action were also discussed.

Macdonald Critchley (1965) preferred the word "corporeal awareness." He said, "this term is expressly chosen in preference to the conventional 'body image' and 'body schema' which fail to indicate the combined properties of a concept and a percept" (p. 68).

As indicated from the above references, medical specialists and psychologists in the last twenty-five years have shown a renewed interest in research and theories concerning the self. Ruth Wylie (1961) extensively reviewed the recent empirical literature. She used the term "self concept" to mean the individual who is known to himself and suggested that psychologists interested in the self concept area conduct more relevant, well-controlled, scientific research. She said, "it is true that personality theories which stress the self have addressed themselves to important unanswered questions concerning human behavior. However, the empirical evidence supporting the theories is limited in proportion to the effort expended" (p. 322-3).

Hodge Eagleson (1966) said that when clinicians treated patients whose body images were very different from their true body status, the concept of "body" had to be exploited to the good of the patient. He also indicated that whenever there was going to be a substantial change in the physical status of the patient, the clinicians had to be extremely gentle, understanding, and analytically oriented, since time was needed for the patient's body image to adjust to real bodily changes. Eagleson felt that the attitude a patient had about his body was important in his recovery and in the acceptance of his limitations.

Self Concept and Speech

STUTTERERS. In a number of publications related to the treatment of individuals who stutter, the importance of improving a person's self concept as a part of the therapeutic situation was stressed. Leading authorities in the speech field, writing in a Speech Foundation of America publication (1960), stated, "With many people who stutter, a major part of their problem seems to involve a disturbed concept of themselves as being different from other people" (pp. 27-28).

According to Ruth Clark and Joseph Fitzpatrick (1962), the behavior of stutterers was influenced by their body images (self concepts). The investigators described stuttering as a psychological experience related to the stutterers' feelings and attitudes toward their own bodies. Stuttering appeared to be a subjective encounter that reflected the mental representation the persons had of their "selves" or bodies. The stutterers' reactions were related to attitudes, memories, feelings, and to the fairly stable characteristics they had regarding themselves and their places in society.

LARYNGECTOMEES. In a study by Clark (1968), self concepts of a group of laryngectomized individuals were ascertained by several different tests following surgery. The laryngectomees were evaluated again when they began to participate in a group of persons with similar problems. It appeared that, in spite of the many severe problems posed by the removal of the larynx and the immediate and devastating effect of complete loss of natural speech, the laryngectomees appeared to have good mental attitudes. This attitude was attained in spite of the facts that (1) the members of the group were over fifty years of age, (2) there was a chance that cancer might recur, (3) employment possibilities were limited, and (4) the natural ability to communicate orally had been lost. It was theorized that the group support of individuals who had encountered the same problem enabled the majority of the members to face an irreversible situation and make an acceptable adjustment to it. It seemed that a realistic self concept had been established and good mental hygiene achieved by most of the laryngectomees.

LEARNING FACILITATION

Burl Grey and Gene England (1969) stated that "human behavior can be explained in terms of the laws of learning and that changes in human behavior can be affected by proper application of the principles of learning and conditioning" (p. iii).

Learning Theory

Learning theory explains behavior through the relationship between the environment or external stimuli and the response. "The learning theorist divides the psychological world into stimuli, responses, and the relationships between these two classes of phenomena that develop from experience. The relationships include habit strength, stimulus generalization, response extinction, and response-contingent reinforcement . . . stimuli may be proprioceptive or exteroceptive; responses may be emotional or instrumental; and reinforcement may be positive or negative" (Brutten and Shoemaker, 1967, p. 7). Learning theory emphasizes behavior, antecedents, and consequences, and does not classify people into character types. The same learning principles apply to maladaptive and adaptive behavior.

Behavior Modification

In the field of speech pathology and audiology, numerous books and articles in professional journals encompass behavioral terms in their titles.

Charles Van Riper (1970) in "Conditioning in Stuttering Therapy" said, "Since its early beginning, our profession has been built on a foundation of learning theory, and modern behavior modification constitutes only the latest storey of the edifice. . . . We have always dealt with problems of learning and unlearning. Our basic function has been to modify communicative behaviors so that the people who come to us would be able to communicate more effectively" (p. 9).

William H. Perkins (1971) in *Speech Pathology, An Applied Behavioral Science,* described various ways of measuring changes in behavior. He said, "What started as a drizzle of operant conditioning studies with the early work of B. F. Skinner . . . soon reached deluge proportions; and the monsoon season has now spread to speech pathology. The concept may even prove to be one of the very few solid rocks on which speech pathology and all other behavioral sciences can be built" (p. 30).

The terms *operant conditioning, behavior modification, reinforcement therapy, behavior therapy, desensitization,* and *learning theory* are frequently encountered in the literature. These terms do not represent new approaches. Indeed, the idea that organisms will avoid "painful" stimuli and will seek "enjoyable" events has been known for a long time. The "pleasure-pain" principle of Freud is an example.

Even though the psychologists have spearheaded the development of modern behavioral modification, speech clinicians have always been behavior therapists. According to Van Riper (1970), the basic concepts and methods of classical and operant conditioning are applied every day in the professional lives of those treating speech, language, voice, and hearing disorders.

The basic principle of all the different techniques used in these approaches is that behavior is a result of its consequences, and as a result of these consequences, the behavior can be strengthened or weakened. Stated simply, reward and punishment serve to regulate behavior.

The reward or pleasure principle of behavior modification or learning theory seems to be confirmed by techniques that incorporate intraoral and extraoral stimulations. That is, the speech-impaired individual can frequently succeed in producing acceptable speech when being assisted by selected, consistent stimulations. As success becomes apparent and articulation skills improve, many parent-child, husband-wife, employer-employee, and client-clinician relationships appear to improve.

Summary Statement

Dittman (1955) provided statements that summarize the rationale and the major portion of research reviewed in this chapter. She postulated that the probable value of sensorimotor techniques lay in one or more of the following processes:

1. It may increase the tonicity of the speech musculature, thus creating a physical climate for speech.
2. The various stimulations may result in a conditioned response, i.e. when a certain pressure is applied, regardless of where it may be or of its neurophysiological relationship to the desired movement, it is conditioned to call out a certain muscular or vocal response.
3. The gross movement patterns with jaw activity possibly produce proprioceptive excitation and aid in training in positional sense.
4. The intense visual and auditory training which accompanies the kinesthetic cues is quite possibly of as much or more value in the actual learning process than the majority of the movements and pressure stimulations.
5. The psychological benefit derived from the close physical contact and undivided attention of the therapist is in all probability an outstanding factor in the motivation of speech in this particular method (p. 132).

Chapter 3

HISTORICAL OVERVIEW

- DEVELOPMENT AND REFINEMENT OF THE MOTO-KINESTHETIC METHOD
  - Edna Hill Young
  - Sara Stinchfield Hawk
  - Further Dissemination of the Technique
- INTRAORAL DEVICES
  - Plastic Palate
  - Zonds
  - Electrical Stimulation
  - Intraoral Tactile Monitoring Systems
  - Dillydots®
  - Intraoral Training Guides
  - Tongue Blades
- OTHER STIMULATION SYSTEMS
  - Visual Tactile System
  - Vibrotactile Stimulation
  - Kinesthetic Cues
  - Visual-Auditory Cues
  - Proprioceptive Neuromuscular Technique

DEVELOPMENT AND REFINEMENT OF THE MOTO-KINESTHETIC METHOD

Edna Hill Young

At ninety years of age, Edna Hill Young, originator of the Moto-kinesthetic Method, was still helping persons overcome their speech problems. She was especially dedicated to young children who needed to learn muscular control essential to clear speech.

Edna Hill Young became interested in the field of speech correction when, at the age of fifteen, she began analyzing her own speech. She had already overcome a speech defect, but she found that "her mouth tired easily when she spoke." She observed the speech movements of others, retrained her own speech muscles, and began to help others acquire more comfortable speech patterns.

Initially, Young opened a school of speech and a clinic in Minneapolis, Minnesota. Upon invitation, she opened similar schools and clinics in Los Angeles, California, and Denver, Colorado. Rockefeller Foundation and Marshall Field grants assisted her in research related to the Moto-kinesthetic Technique.

One of the greatest satisfactions in life for Edna Hill Young was being able to assist her husband regain his speech after a stroke left him aphasic. Throughout her lifetime, her students and clients responded to her warm and dynamic personality. Because of her gentle and reassuring manner, many children with whom she worked called her "Mother Young."

Edna Hill Young received an Honorary Doctor of Pedagogy degree from Hastings College in 1944, the Honors of the California Speech and Hearing Association in 1964, and was made a Fellow and Life Member of the American Speech and Hearing Association.

Several of Young's articles appeared in the *Journal of Speech and Hearing Disorders,* including: "The Moto-kinesthetic Method of Speech Training" in 1940, "A Personal Experience with Speech" in 1958, and "The Moto-kinesthetic Approach to the Prevention of Speech Defects, Including Stuttering" in 1965.

In 1951, Edna Hill Young made a motion picture of the Moto-kinesthetic Technique. She was assisted by Ruth Van Tine, R. Edwin Shutts, Richard Woellhof, and Richard Winchester. She wrote the following notes to go with the film:

> The big essential to success in the use of this method is that the teacher learns the technique thoroughly, so that she may get the results which skill can produce. Such skill comes only through persistent practice.
>
> This kind of help is useful in therapy whenever changes in movement are involved. It may also be used in cooperation with other techniques, as in cleft-palate cases. It is especially needed for the severely handicapped groups, the speechless child, whose help should come earlier than it usually does, to prevent permanent handicap. It has been surprising to me to see the ease with which the child from eighteen to thirty months learns movements through the feel of correct patterns. It seems to be the age especially right for learning through the kinesthetic.
>
> I have seen certain cerebral palsied cases of varying ages greatly improved through the application of this method, adjusted to the needs of the individual case. I have seen certain adult aphasics re-enact their former habitual movements, bringing words after feeling the lost pattern as applied by another.

> Care must be observed not to plunge into the use of these techniques with a new subject until previous preparation has been made. The psychological aspects of training, the understanding of human beings, and of the individual case, is fully as important to success as the manipulations.
>
> In closing, I hope that this film will go out and be a real value to you, who are engaged in the sometimes wearisome task of speech correction (p. 39).

The manual in which Edna Hill Young made the above comments was written by Ruth M. Clark and Ruth Van Tine (1947), with a foreword by Richard Woellhof.

Before Edna Hill Young died, research was beginning in oral sensation and discrimination, and in the relationships of kinesthesia, touch-pressure, and proprioception.

Sara Stinchfield Hawk

Sara Stinchfield Hawk was the first *person* and first *woman* to receive a doctorate with a psychology-speech major. The degree was awarded in 1922, at the University of Wisconsin.

Sara S. Hawk wrote "Moto-kinesthetic Training for Children with Speech Handicaps," *Journal of Speech Disorders,* 1942.

In 1938, Sara Stinchfield Hawk and Edna Hill Young collaborated in introducing the Moto-kinesthetic Method of articulation therapy. They stressed the development of correct movement patterns and required the clinician to manipulate or stimulate the articulators.

Stinchfield [Hawk] and Young authored *Children with Delayed and Defective Speech: Moto-Kinesthetic Factors in Their Training* in 1938. Young and Hawk wrote *Moto-Kinesthetic Speech Training* in 1955.

Hawk contributed greatly to the refinement of the Moto-kinesthetic approach to speech therapy before she died.

Young and Hawk (1955) observed that ". . . the manipulation of muscles should rarely be attempted in the first contacts of teacher and patient. Whatever period of time is necessary should be allowed for getting acquainted, leading gradually to the thought of speech. Without the correct approach psychologically, the manipulations may fail, but without added help through the manipulations, psychology cannot do alone, in many cases, what the combined therapies can do together. . . ." (p. 11).

Further Dissemination of the Technique

In a 1974 publication, Ronald K. Sommers and Ann R. Kane described the stimulation or manipulation of the speech muscles as a means to help a respondent understand the manner in which the articulators work individually and in coordination in the production of sounds. They described stimulation by touch as an attempt to develop kinesthetic patterns through movement and pressure. They indicated that when the stimulator said the sound or word, auditory patterns were established simultaneously with the manipulation and that visual cues occurred as the respondent observed the stimulator's speech pattern.

A number of Mrs. Young's students disseminated her technique. Clark (1962) wrote "Application of the Moto-Kinesthetic Method in the Speech Clinic," and prepared a manual in cooperation with Van Tine (1949) entitled *Directions for Stimulating Speech by the Moto-Kinesthetic Method.* This manual was mimeographed and was used widely by persons studying at the University of Denver.

As a part of doctoral level studies at the Universidad Nacional de Mexico, the Moto-kinesthetic Method stimulations were translated into Spanish in 1951, by Gwenyth R. Vaughn. The material in Spanish was directed toward the training of teachers of the deaf in Mexico. The format used for the Spanish translation is the one utilized for the Speech Facilitation stimulation units in this text.

For a number of years, Sylvester Clifford of the University of South Dakota has been teaching courses and presenting workshops in the Moto-kinesthetic Method. He also assisted in developing a film to be used in the teaching of Moto-kinesthetic procedures.

Lily Tjomsland (1968) studied with Young and later with Clifford. She produced a book that included several of the Moto-kinesthetic stimulations.

George Shaffer was a student of Young's and later taught the Moto-kinesthetic Method at Purdue University.

Additional articles are listed in the *References* (Cable, 1945; Clark, 1962; Flowers, 1966; Hahn, 1939 and 1940; Stinchfield Hawk, 1935, 1937, 1938, 1939 a & b, 1941, 1942, 1944 a & b, 1964; Pfoff, 1940; Travis, 1940; Young, 1945, 1967).

INTRAORAL DEVICES

Plastic Palate

Gerhardt H. Breckwoldt (1948) utilized artificial palates for teaching a deaf boy the visual processes of articulation that otherwise were not visible to the eye. In order to do this, plastic palates were made for the boy and for Breckwoldt. The thin plastic sheet exactly fit the hard palate and part of the soft palate. A white powder such as magnesium carbonate or powdered sugar was used to rub the dark inner surface so lingual contact would be revealed.

After the artificial palates were pressed into place in their mouths, the boy and his professor articulated. When the palates were removed, the patterns of the articulation were observable. By transferring the pattern to line diagrams drawn in exact proportion to the artificial palate, a palatogram, or picture of the articulation of the sound, was easily studied. Measurements of the spaces touched by the tongue provided additional information beyond the visual cues shown by the diagram.

When the sounds were articulated correctly, almost identical patterns were produced by both the boy and his professor. The sounds the boy produced indistinctly were in sharp contrast to the pattern of his professor. Sometimes the boy demonstrated a direct inversion of the correct position.

Zonds

In Russia, according to Clark (1961), the use of oral stimulation for correcting speech problems was an accepted part of the general treatment program entitled "defectology." Wire devices called *Zonds* were utilized in speech correction classes. A Zond was used to force the tongue into a prescribed position for the production of a particular sound. Each sound had a different Zond. Only one sound at a time was subjected to treatment. The Director of Logopedics in the Institute of Defectology in Moscow stated that he felt that Zonds were an important aid in speech therapy and that a child could be cured of his articulation mistakes in two days' time with their help.

Electrical Stimulation

Richard C. Grossman and James F. Bosma (1963) developed a thin palatal prosthesis with a relay activator circuit and a standard laboratory stimulator. This prosthesis was used to provide electrical stimulation for persons deficient in oral surface perception.

The relay circuit was completed when the tongue made contact with a trigger electrode on the lingual surface of the prosthesis. This contact activated the stimulator which provided direct current pulses of controlled duration, frequency, and voltage to a stimulating electrode on the palatal surface of the prosthesis. The stimulation continued as long as the tongue remained in contact with the trigger electrode. A cathode ray oscilloscope served as a monitor of the stimulus. The duration of each tongue-to-palate contact was indicated by a small electric lamp. The lamp also served as a reinforcement of the electrical stimulus in conditioning the subject to the supplemented sensory experience.

Intraoral Tactile Monitoring System

According to some authors, "Utilization of an oral-tactile approach may be more suitable as a rehabilitative method" (Fucci and Robertson, 1971, p. 714). McDonald (1967) suggested the remediation of articulatory disturbances through the heightening of an individual's awareness of kinesthetic and tactile cues by asking him to describe the various parts of the mouth that were touching each other and the direction and movement of the tongue during a particular production.

In addition to the studies mentioned above, several other authors have written about proprioceptive, tactile, and kinesthetic feedback in treatment of persons with communicative disorders (Eggermont, 1960; Rutherford and McCall, 1967; Filter, 1974; Darley, 1975).

Robert S. Ringel, Anne H. B. Putnam, and William N. Williams (1974) utilized a therapy program to work with children with defective tactile monitoring systems. These programs consisted of three phases:

A. Phase I:
   1. Place object in client's mouth. Are the objects the same or different? How are they the same or different?
   2. Look at the objects; put them back in the mouth.
   3. Draw a picture of the objects.

B. Phase II:
   1. Stimulate the oral cavity with swabs of cotton going over contact areas saying: "This is where contact will be made."
   2. Use phonetic placement.
   3. Have client make clay model of oral structure; place pegs where contact is made.

C. Phase III:
   1. Stimulate.
   2. Discuss points of contact (p. 5).

Studies have shown that therapy directed at oral sensory training did result in improvement of defective articulation (Wilhelm, 1966; Ruscello and Lass, 1972).

Dillydots®

In addition to the usual verbal explanation for physical placement of the articulators and observation of speech positions in the mirror, the developers of Grape Dillydots felt that a "tasty reward" helped achieve greater motivation. Dillydots (1976) were recommended for teaching the lingua-alveolar sounds.

Intraoral Training Aid

An intraoral training aid for the speech rehabilitation of laryngectomy patients was developed by Jack Light, Sidney I. Silverman, and Lawrence Garfinkel (1976). It was hypothesized that the prosthesis provided (1) heightened tactile cues afforded by an increased tactile-kinesthetic sense, (2) modification of the oral space volume, and (3) success in producing better acoustic products as the result of the reinforcement technique.

Tongue Blades

Clinicians have long employed tongue blades to stimulate intraoral sensitivity. The tongue blades are used to push back, lower, and curl the edges of the tongue as well as to indicate the point of contact between the tongue and the other articulators.

OTHER STIMULATION SYSTEMS

Visual Tactile System

Zaliouk (1954) prepared a "visual-tactile system of phonetic symbolization" to be used with deaf children. He employed two categories of symbols—static and dynamic. The hard palate, tongue, teeth, and lips were represented by the static symbols; movement was represented by the dynamic symbols. The system sought to use accessible afferent pathways of the tactile, kinesthetic, and visual senses. The importance of maintaining a structural "Gestalt" in the flow of spoken language was considered to be crucial. Zaliouk felt that such a system should (1) cover every area of applied phonetics, (2) be easily adaptable to any language, (3) be built on sound and well-established physiological data, (4) be simple in conception and easy to use, (5) be applicable to a wide variety of pathological conditions, (6) be appropriate for use with persons of different ages, and (7) provide graphic representation so simple that it could be easily grasped by clinician and client.

Vibrotactile Stimulation

Kal Telage and Donald Fucci (1973) described the development of vibrotactile equipment and summarized a number of studies concerned with the rationale and methods to obtain thresholds of oral tactile sensitivity. The studies included threshold responses of normal and abnormal speakers to vibrotactile stimulation and described research on the lower lip as well as the tongue.

In speculating about the diagnostic and therapeutic significance of vibrotactile stimulation as a clinical tool for speech pathologists, they concluded that thresholds could be obtained on the tactile sensibility of the tongue as well as thresholds on hearing. Telage and Fucci pointed out that the diagnostician could determine whether or not a patient was "hard of feeling" as well as "hard of hearing." Utilizing vibrotactile thresholds, they said, would provide diagnostically "a more complete picture of the tactile sensory feedback system used in speech production" (p. 446).

The above authors have not determined whether or not oral-tactile information would be useful in therapeutic procedures. Telage and Fucci felt that the information gained from vibrotactile testing would be helpful in evaluation but that Moto-kinesthetic and phonetic placement techniques would be used more extensively for treatment. They felt that the latter method provided direct tactile experience to the major articulators used in speech and that "perhaps the speech pathologists would also develop techniques for tactile sensory rehabilitation which would incorporate drills or other clinical procedures to enable patients to make better use of residual oral sensory capabilities" (p. 446).

Telage and Fucci suggested that many children who are now thought to have "functional" articulation problems may in reality have oral-tactile sensory deficits. They proposed that if these children were properly diagnosed, rehabilitative procedures could be instituted that would focus on the oral sensory problem. They also listed several steps needed to make vibrotactile methodology a clinical success.

The literature reports that many teachers and clinicians working with deaf children use touch to give cues concerning vocalization and resonation. Contacts with sounding boards, pianos, diaphragms, balloons, and bone conductor vibrators and other tactile coders supplement auditory and visual cues.

Kinesthetic Cues

Tongue and lip exercises have been used to assist persons in identifying the movements integral to articulation of speech sounds. Other bodily movements have been combined with the speech movements for reinforcement through the kinesthetic sense.

The usefulness of using touch and body movement as a means of conveying information to deaf, blind, and deaf-blind children has been demonstrated (Chalfant and Scheffelin, 1969).

Only a few teaching methods have emphasized touch (tactile) and body movement for teaching normally seeing and hearing children (Montessori, 1912; Fernald, 1939; Strauss and Lehtinen, 1947; and Gillingham and Stillman, 1960).

Visual-Auditory Cues

Most of the speech sounds have poor visibility and many have low acoustic power. When acoustic input is reduced or distorted, the learning of accurate articulation becomes more difficult. If articulation defects are present, evaluation of tactile, kinesthetic, and proprioceptive channels may provide important information.

Some clinicians have supported the theory of unisensory stimulation; others have preferred the auditory-visual combination for teaching hearing-impaired children. As diagnostic techniques become more sophisticated, it may be possible to identify the sensory modalities best suited for each person.

Proprioceptive Neuromuscular Facilitation Techniques

Annette A. May and Douglas A. Hudgens (1977) suggested the application of specific neuromuscular facilitation procedures in the management of persons with dysarthria. Techniques included (1) icing, (2) stroking, (3) positioning, (4) controlled response elicitation, and (5) other specific activities.

Linda S. Remblisz and Sabra A. Gribin (1977) developed techniques for treating children and adults with dysarthria. Their approach included procedures to strengthen (1) lingual, labial, and palatal muscles; (2) diminish tongue thrust and drooling; (3) develop feeding and drinking skills; and (4) improve articulatory skills.

SECTION II

Speech Facilitation Procedures

INTRODUCTION

SPEECH FACILITATION may be utilized as a primary or supplementary technique for the improvement of articulatory skills. Speech Facilitation assists in the teaching and learning of articulatory functions through the use of extraoral manipulations and cues, and phonodental guides and intraoral cues.

Speech Facilitation is not intended for the refinement of speech. The manipulations and cues are designed to create for the respondent an awareness of articulatory movements and placements. Conditioning, feedback, and reinforcement contribute to the ultimate incorporation of improved articulatory patterns into functional speech. The technique lends itself to multisensory and unisensory approaches.

Articulatory impairments that occur singly, or in concert with other disordered aspects of speech, generally respond well to the stimulations of Speech Facilitation. Articulatory problems related to hearing losses, orofacial abnormalities, and neurological deficits or disorders are usually amenable to treatment through the utilization of extraoral manipulations, phonodental guides, and cues.

Speech Facilitation is a treatment plan that helps persons with articulatory disorders to (1) correct laggard sounds in their articulatory patterns, (2) approximate the position of a sound through imitation, when the sound productions are brittle and need stabilization before reinsertion, (3) improve articulatory skills that are severely impaired, and (4) maintain functional articulation skills when speech sounds are deteriorating.

It is important that the person utilizing the manipulations, guides, and cues be not only a competent clinician but also a skilled practitioner of Speech Facilitation. If supportive personnel is utilized, careful supervision by an experienced clinician is necessary.

Purpose of Speech Facilitation

The purpose of Speech Facilitation is three-fold: (1) to clarify and amplify the original instructions for the Moto-kinesthetic stimulations, (2) to furnish additional details for those stimulations, and (3) to describe the production and placement of the Speech Facilitation phonodental guides.

The intent of this volume is to put the extraoral manipulations and intraoral guides of Speech Facilitation into a clinical-scientific perspective based on the *State of the Art* as described in Section I.

Section II Organization

Chapter 4 describes the application of the Speech Facilitation extraoral manipulations and extraoral cues. It provides background information related to each Stimulation Unit and defines the terms used in Speech Facilitation.

Chapter 5 discusses the preparation and placement of the phonodental guides and the use of intraoral cues. The International Dental Federation Tooth Numbering System is used to indicate the placement of the phonodental guides and intraoral cues.

Chapter 4

APPLICATION OF THE EXTRAORAL MANIPULATIONS

- DEFINITION OF SPEECH FACILITATION TERMS
  - Stimulator
  - Respondent
  - Manipulation
- SYMBOL SYSTEMS
- TOPOGRAPHICAL RELATIONSHIPS OF PHONEME PRODUCTION
- SPEECH FACILITATION PRINCIPLES
  - Rapport
  - Position and Movement
  - Timing
  - Rate
  - Pressure
  - Duration
  - Stress
  - Sensory Stimuli
- Additional Application Suggestions
  - Initiation of Sound
  - Stimulation of Sounds or Syllables
  - Similarities and Differences
  - Dialectal Considerations
  - Seating of Respondent During Stimulations
    - Moto-kinesthetic Technique
    - Speech Facilitation
  - Target Phoneme Order
- MANIPULATION MODELS
  - Finger and Hand Format
  - Finger and Hand Cues
  - Face and Lips Format
- BACKGROUND INFORMATION
- Selected Phoneme Characteristics
  - Developmental Age
  - Frequency of Occurrence of Phonemes
  - Visual Confusion

- Auditory Intelligibility
- Auditory Confusion
- Relative Phonetic Power
- Phonemic Confusion
- Typical Spelling

• PRACTICE MATERIALS

DEFINITION OF SPEECH FACILITATION TERMS

Stimulator

THE TERM *stimulator* refers to the person applying the extraoral manipulations, the finger and hand cues, and phonodental guides.

Respondent

The term *respondent* refers to the persons responding to the stimulations. This term covers the words in common usage such as *patient, client,* and *student.*

Manipulation

According to *Dorland's Illustrated Medical Dictionary* (1965), manipulation means "Skillful or dextrous treatment by hand." In Speech Facilitation, extraoral manipulations are provided through prescribed manual movement, timing, and pressure exerted on the extraoral speech mechanism and accompanying air current of the respondent by someone qualified to do so.

SYMBOL SYSTEMS

Several symbol systems are used in Speech Facilitation so that persons who are familiar with any one of the systems can easily interpret the identification symbols used in the Stimulation Units. The phonetic symbol is always followed by a representative word in parentheses. The word is for identification purposes only and not necessarily for use in stimulating the phoneme.

The International Phonetic Alphabet Symbols, with slight modifications, are taken from *And So We Speak* by Johnnye Akin (1958, pp. 10 and 85). Some of the IPA symbols have been recently modified by the linguists. The changes are not used in Speech Facilitation.

The symbols familiar to dictionary users come from *Webster's New Collegiate Dictionary* (1965, p. 15a). For persons involved in education of the deaf, the Thorndike Symbols from the *Thorndike-Barnhardt Comprehensive Dictionary* (1951) are included as are the Northampton Chart Symbols from *Formation and Development of Elementary English Sounds* (Yale, 1946, pp. 10 and 11).

TOPOGRAPHICAL RELATIONSHIPS OF PHONEME PRODUCTION

Topographical relationships are described in terms of the mandible; lips; tongue tip, body, and sides; air stream; nasal port; and vocal folds.

At the beginning of each Section, figures give representative positions of the tongue for the vowels, diphthongs, and consonants.

SPEECH FACILITATION PRINCIPLES

The principles underlying the application of the extraoral stimulations of Speech Facilitation include:

1. establishment of stimulator-respondent rapport,
2. teaching of position and movement for each phoneme,
3. utilization of timing, rate, pressure, duration, and stress, and
4. addition or exclusion of sensory stimuli.

Rapport

Professionals who incorporate the extraoral manipulations and cues and intraoral guides of Speech Facilitation need to explain the rationale to the respondents so they will be prepared for the various forms of stimulation.

Some persons enjoy being "touched." It is thought that the psychology of touching persons in treatment often offers comfort and promotes understanding between stimulator and respondent.

Position and Movement

The positions and movements suggested for the phonemes in the Stimulation Units conform with those found in most phonetic texts.

The finger placement for the manipulations is indicated by numbers on the Manipulation Models. The stimulator may make some modifications in finger placement and movement, if the changes facilitate the desired response.

Timing

The stimulator should not try to hurry the manipulations. A rhythm must be established so the respondent will know when to expect the stimulation. The extraoral manipulation should be made with all deliberateness. The stimulator should not apply the stimulation until the respondent is prepared to receive it.

It is usually desirable to pause before and after the stimulation of the target phoneme. Delay in blending the target sound with the other sounds in the syllable or word is reduced as the person learns to synthesize the adjacent phonemes. Rhythm must be maintained, no matter what the length of the pause. A longer interval is often utilized in the initial stimulation. It is gradually shortened until it is ultimately eliminated as the respondent learns to integrate the phoneme into the syllable or word.

Rate

A *slower rate* in the stimulation permits a lengthening of the target phoneme. The stimulator may need to utilize *holding time* during the manipulation in order for the respondent to *register the feel* of the articulatory position and movement.

After the learning period, any tendency of a respondent to produce the target phoneme in an exaggerated manner should be corrected. The timing and rhythm of "normal" speech should be constantly kept in mind by the stimulator. The tempo and pattern of the stimulator's own speech may serve as a guide.

Pressure

The pressure exerted by all of the fingers involved in the manipulations should be equal. ***Increased pressure*** by the fingers not only signals but seems to stimulate phonation. The pressure should not be so great, however, that the stimulation becomes uncomfortable for the respondent or detracts from the sensation that is intended to stimulate a particular articulatory position and movement.

Duration

Both duration and pressure provide cues signaling phonation. The stimulatory position should be held long enough for vocalization to be initiated in the voiced phonemes.

Stress

If *stress* is shifted, production of some syllables becomes more difficult for some respondents. The use of repetition as in di-syllabic words may help overcome this difficulty.

Sensory Stimuli

The extraoral and/or intraoral stimulations are usually combined with auditory and visual stimuli. The latter are generally presented prior to the extraoral or intraoral stimuli. They are often accompanied by an explanation of the desired articulatory placements and movements. All of the selected stimuli are then presented simultaneously. If auditory and/or visual stimuli are not to be utilized, the manipulations, cues, and guides are used alone. When visual stimulation is included, the respondent may look at the stimulator directly prior to or during the stimulation. It is sometimes awkward to apply the extraoral manipulation when the respondent is directly facing the stimulator. The visual and/or auditory cues are usually repeated simultaneously with the extraoral manipulation.

Additional Application Suggestions

Initiation of Sound

If a respondent has difficulty in initiating sound, it may be the result of faulty coordination of respiration, phonation, or articulation. Pressing the hand just below the rib cage at the midline usually overcomes the air flow difficulty. The /h/ (*h*oe) may be used to initiate any response. The /h/ (*h*oe) may be faded subsequently.

Stimulation of Sounds or Syllables

For phonemes in the initial position, the syllable is the speech unit of choice. If the person is unable to move easily from one sound to another, a single vowel, or a single consonant, often accompanied by an unstimulated schwa /ə/ (sof*a*), may be taught. As soon as the ability to produce one-syllable responses is stabilized, repetitive disyllable words such as *mama, papa,* and *bye-bye* may be initiated.

The stimulator does not provide any manipulations for the sounds in the syllable or word that the respondent can produce correctly. For example, if the respondent can produce the first two sounds in the word *dog,* but omits or distorts the final sound, the topographical stimulation is given only for that final sound. The stimulation for the final sound is given with proper rhythm after the person has produced the first two sounds. The final stimulation should be applied in an unhurried manner and may be considerably delayed at first. The pause between the articulation of the first two sounds and the final sound is then gradually reduced until the sounds are produced in a "normal" manner and rate.

Similarities and Differences

For respondents or supportive personnel who do not have a previous background in the production of speech sounds, pointing out the similarities and differences is usually helpful; for example, being made aware that many of the consonants are similar, except for the voiced or voiceless quality of a pair of sounds. The manipulations for most of these paired sounds are similar except when (1) greater pressure and longer duration indicates phonation for the voiced consonant, and (2) lesser pressure and shorter duration signals the voiceless counterpart. A quick release of the manipulation signals plosiveness in the voiceless plosive sounds.

Dialectal Considerations

Phoneticians and linguists recognize variant pronunciations in the United States. Because of the mobility of the population and mass media, however, the dialectal regions are not well defined. Although the stimulations presented in the *Manual* are based on pronunciations commonly found in standard dictionaries, some adjustments in the placement, movement, and timing of the manipulations are necessary in order to incorporate regional differences when desired.

Seating of Respondent During Stimulations

Moto-kinesthetic Technique. During the application of the Moto-kinesthetic Technique, Edna Hill Young provided a table on which the respondents lay on their backs. The table was of a comfortable working height for the stimulators who were seated at the side of the table.

As additional clinicians began to utilize the Technique, many persons with articulatory disorders received therapy in the public schools or similar settings, and it was not possible to arrange for a therapy space in which a table could be installed.

Speech Facilitation. The Speech Facilitation manipulations have been designed so they may be applied satisfactorily with the stimulator and respondent seated in adjacent chairs, facing in opposite directions.

The chairs of the stimulator and respondent are placed side-by-side with the face of the respondent within easy reach of the stimulator. The stimulator is seated so that the preferred hand is next to the respondent, thus facilitating its use in the extraoral manipulations. When phonodental guides are used singly or in combination with the extraoral manipulations, the seating is arranged so that the hand holding the phonodental guide does not interfere with the hand applying the manipulations.

Before applying the manipulations, the stimulator places the respondent's head in the optimal position for applying the manipulation. This may mean that the respondent's head is turned slightly away from the stimulator. When the manipulations are being applied, the respondent's head is not allowed to move backward or downward. When a downward head movement does occur, the palm of the hand of the stimulator is placed against the respondent's forehead. Enough pressure is exerted to hold the respondent's head steady. If the opposite occurs and the respondent's head tips backward, pressure of the stimulator's hand against the back of the head reduces movement during application of the manipulation. If the respondent does not relax sufficiently

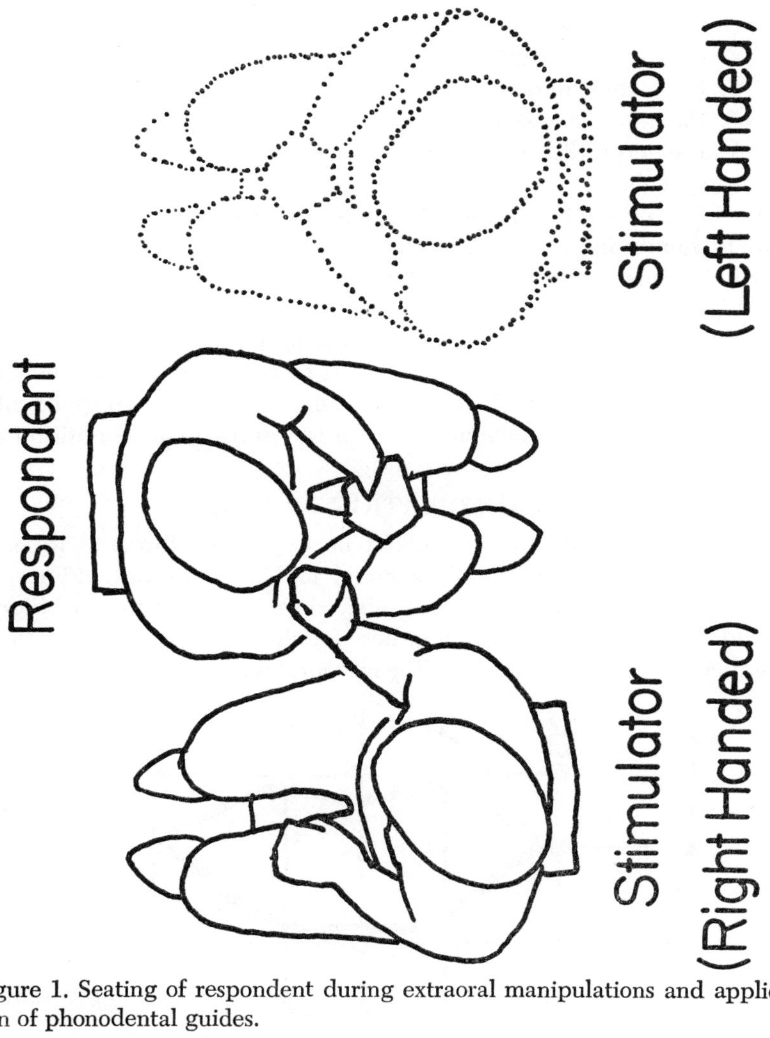

Figure 1. Seating of respondent during extraoral manipulations and application of phonodental guides.

to allow the mandible to be lowered, the stimulator should shake the mandible gently with a side-to-side motion.

Target Phoneme Order

The order in which the defective speech sounds are taught is usually established on one of the following bases:

1. the most easily stimulated by the Speech Facilitation technique,
2. the one articulated correctly in one-or-more words that can be modified,

3. the most visible and/or audible, or most easily imitated,
4. the most easily articulated,
5. the earliest in developmental order,
6. the most commonly occurring in the language, or
7. the most disturbing to the intelligibility of the respondent's speech.

In Speech Facilitation, the Stimulation Units are self-contained and may be taught in any order. Chapter 7 discusses the suggested practice order. Sounds are most easily taught when the extreme vowels are combined with the most visible consonants.

Trainees should first practice the manipulations in the initial position. When teaching articulatory skills to respondents with defective sounds, the stimulator should determine whether the respondent is able to produce the phoneme better in the initial or final position and begin teaching the sound accordingly.

MANIPULATION MODELS

The Manipulation models consist of (1) a lips format with numbered points (Figure 2), (2) a finger and hand format (Figure 3), and (3) a face format with numbered points (Figure 4). Figures 3 and 4 are designed with numbered points that correspond to the numbers given in directions for the extraoral manipulations.

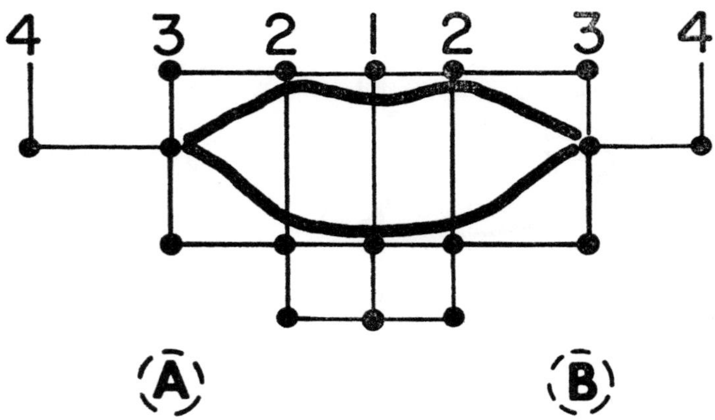

Figure 2. Manipulation model: lips format.

Lips Format

Figure 2 provides a Manipulation Model of the lips. These numbered models of the lips are placed next to the instructions for the extraoral manipulations in each Stimulation Unit. This model may be used to practice the extraoral manipulations before they are used with respondents.

Finger and Hand Format

In the manipulations, the following terms are assigned the fingers: *thumb, index, middle, ring,* and *little.* (See Figure 3.) The numbering system for the manipulations makes the hands interchangeable.

The *thumb* and *middle* finger are utilized in the starting position. This selection leaves the *index* finger available for cueing or manipulating and the *little* finger for signaling phonation.

Finger and Hand Cues

Finger and hand cues consist of (1) placing a finger on the side of the nose to signal nasalization, (2) touching the larynx with a finger to signal phonation, or (3) pressing the palm of one hand just below the respondent's rib cage at the midline to signal breath expiration. In the latter, the degree of hand pressure is used to activate a sudden or a gradual expiration of breath. If the respondent holds his hand

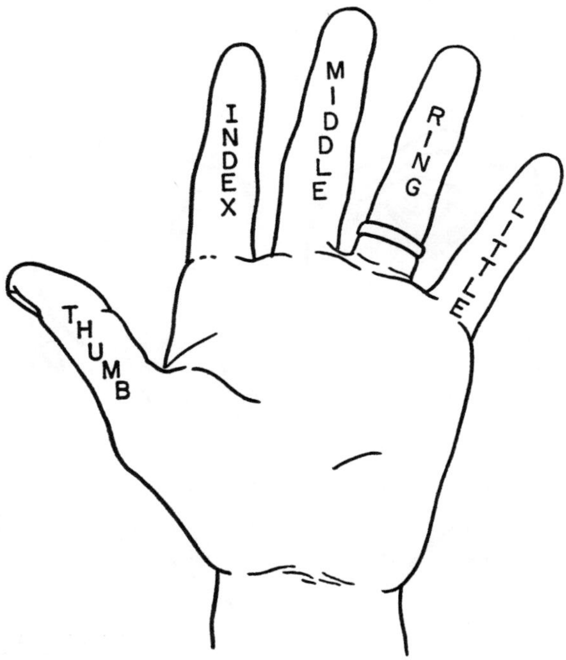

Figure 3. Manipulation model: finger and hand format.

in front of his own mouth, or that of the stimulator, the timing, length, and force of the breath may be monitored.

Face and Lips Format

The face format consists of the upper lip, mid-lip, lower lip, mid-chin, and sub-chin points intersecting with lines numbered from one through four. The side of the nose and the larynx are also identified as points to be used for finger cueing. (See Figure 4.)

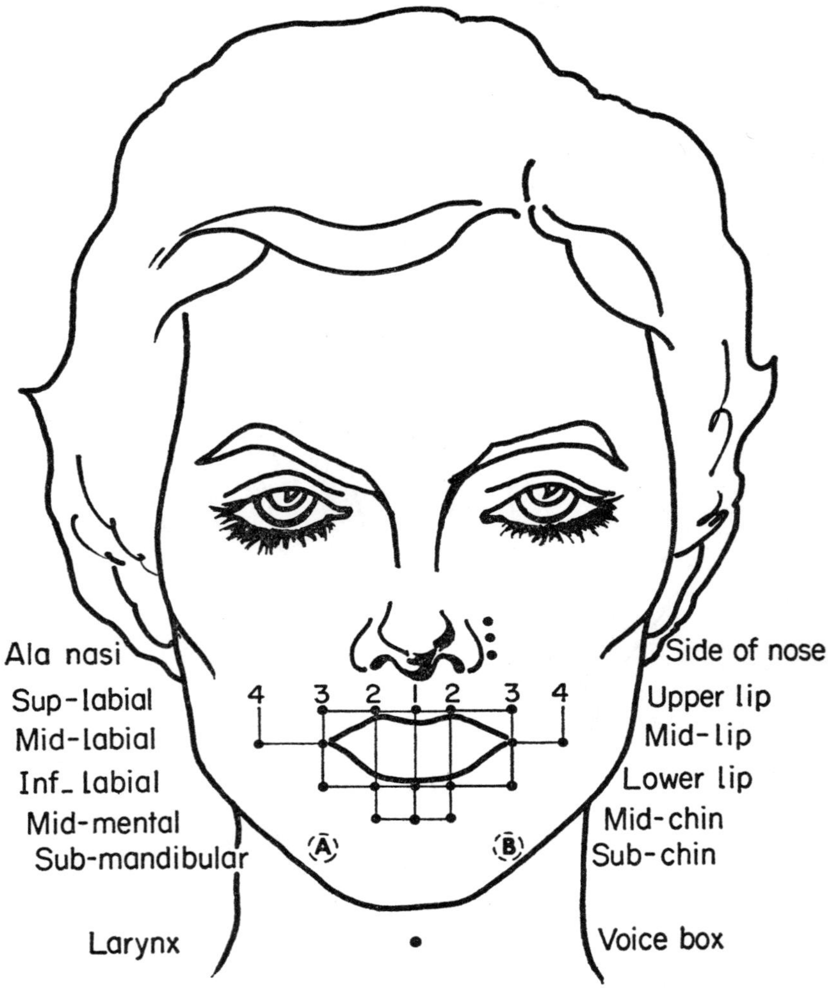

Figure 4. Manipulation model: face format.

BACKGROUND INFORMATION

Selected Phoneme Characteristics

Selected characteristics are listed for each phoneme. The information includes: (1) developmental age at which each sound usually appears, (2) frequency of occurrence of each phoneme in the English language, (3) visual intelligibility, (4) likely visual confusion in attempts at speech reading, (5) auditory intelligibility in mild-to-severe hearing impairments, (6) sounds that may present problems of auditory confusion, (7) relative phonetic power of the phonemes, (8) sounds that are closely related and may result in phonemic confusion, and (9) typical spelling of each sound. The background information is placed prior to the practice materials. The practice materials are located at the end of each Stimulation Unit.

Developmental Age

According to Templin (1957), the relative difficulty of specific sounds is an important consideration in articulation development. Although the importance of age in the relationship between age and acquisition of sounds does not draw forth equal support from all investigators, many clinicians find information concerning developmental age useful.

Each sound that was tested by Templin was reported for the age at which 75 percent of the children produced it correctly. The only sounds of those tested that were not produced correctly by 75 percent of the subjects were *hw-*, *-hw-*, *-tl*, and *-lfth*. The 75 percent level of attainment did not continue consistently for all of the sounds after the earliest age at which it was entered. The sounds that did not conform were *-t*, *-rm*, *-kr*, *br-*, *sm-*, *-rt*, *-ft*, *-mpt*, *pl-*, *l-*, *sp-*, *sn-*, and *-sh-* (1957, p. 51).

The Templin study was in substantial agreement with those made by Beth Wellman and others (1936) and Irene Poole (1934).

Frequency of Occurrence of Phonemes

Charles Hutton (1969) stated that phoneme occurrence was a language variable that influenced visual and auditory intelligibility. Hutton reported J. V. Tobias' (1959) study of the relative occurrence of forty-two phonemes in American English. Of the forty phonemes listed, nine accounted for 50 percent of phoneme occurrence. Hutton pointed out that unfortunately for many hearing-impaired persons, most of the frequently occurring phonemes were those that had the least visual intelligibility.

John Dorn (1974) made a phonetic context analysis of General American consonants and vowels. The phonemes of /p,b,o,ɑ,ɚ/ (*p*ut, *b*oy, *o*bey, l*o*t, sist*er*) were listed in the top nineteen phonemes by Dorn in contrast with Tobias who listed the same phonemes among the lowest twenty-five. Dorn also reported /w, ð/ (*w*e, *th*is) among the lowest of the forty-two pheonemes while Tobias place /ð/ (*th*is) in the highest eight and /w/ (*w*e) in the highest thirteen.

Since the majority of the other sounds were listed by both investigators within the same bracket, the Tobias' study is used as the reference for the background information reported in the Stimulation Units. Hutton (1969) presented a table with the relative percentage rankings of the visual intelligibility of English phonemes according to several studies (Heider and Heider, 1940; Hutton, 1959; O'Neill, 1954; Samuelson, 1943; and Woodward, 1957). A composite of various ratings showed that of the thirty-six phonemes reported by Hutton, twenty of them ranged from 58 to 87 percent visual intelligibility on the composite scale; the remaining sixteen were rated as being visual only 23 to 50 percent of the time. It was apparent that those that were characterized by frontal articulation and labialization were in the upper percentage, while those with mid and back articulation and those that lacked labialization were found, for the most part, in the lower 50 percent of the composite visibility rating scale.

Cornett (1967) developed Cued Speech, a system of hand signs or signals that can be used simultaneously with speech in order to give cues to the speechreader. With the help of Cued Speech, the speechreader can identify obscure and difficult phonemes.

Visual Confusion

According to Hutton (1969, p. 114) the following phonemes were likely to be confused visually.

I.	/p,b,m/	These four confusion groups have strong
II.	/p,w,ʍ/	boundaries. That is, confusion is likely to
III.	/f,v/	occur horizontally, but not vertically.
IV.	/θ,ð/	Identification is high.
V.	(a) /ɔ,ʊ/	This group has very weak boundaries and
	(b) /ɚ,ɑ/	fair identification.
VI.	(a) /t,d,n,l/	These groups have weak boundaries;
	(b) /s,z,ʒ,t,dʒ,j/	horizontal confusions are somewhat more
	(c) /k,g,h/	frequent than vertical confusions. In the
		less proficient lipreader these may be one

		large group. Members from this set are seldom confused with the upper set. Identification is low.
VII.	/ɛ,ɪ,ʌ/	This group has very weak boundaries and low identification. Frequent confusions with other vowel groups occur.

Auditory Intelligibility

Hutton (1969) stated that the extreme vowels and diphthongs were more intelligible than the shorter middle vowels. The nasalized, voiced, longer, and louder consonants were more intelligible than those that were not. The manner of articulation, rather than the place of articulation, was the more important influence in auditory recognition. This was in contrast to visual intelligibility which depended greatly upon place of articulation.

Auditory Confusion

Hutton (1969, p. 128) listed phonemes that are likely to be confused auditorially:

Vowels	Consonants
/u ou/	/m n ŋ/
/au ou/	/w r l/
/i ɪ/	/b d g/
/ou u ɔ/	/p t k h/
/ɔɪ ɔ aɪ æ/	/ʒ z v ð dʒ j/
/eɪ aɪ ɔ/	/ʃ s f θ tʃ/
/ɪ ɛ ʊ ʌ æ/	
/eɪ æ ɛ ɑ/	

Relative Phonetic Power

Harvey Fletcher (1953) gave the relative amount of power of individual speech sounds. The power of the faintest sound was used as a basis of comparison. The most powerful sound was listed as /ɔ/ (*saw*) and the faintest sound as /θ/ (*th*in). The ratio of powers between these two sounds was given as 680.

Phonemic Confusion

Charles Van Riper and John Irwin (1958) stated that errors in the production of speech sounds were generally related acoustically, topographically, or kinesthetically to the target phoneme. These concepts are basic to Speech Facilitation and are reflected in (1) voicing, (2) placement of the articulators, and (4) direction and release of the airstream.

Typical Spelling

The examples of spelling were taken from dictionaries, texts, and other resources commonly in use by educators and speech clinicians.

PRACTICE MATERIALS

Materials for practice are given at the end of each Stimulation Unit. Additional materials may be found at the end of each Section. The Section Practice Materials provide a liberal choice of vowel and consonant combinations. The materials are organized so that similarities and differences are easily apparent. The influence of co-articulation may be noted as the respondent's facility to produce the target phonemes in words and sentences increases. Practice words with adjacent pairs of sounds in which one of the sounds is the defective phoneme and the other is the substituted sound should be avoided until the target phoneme is stabilized. Short sentences are provided for use by the respondent as greater ease in the production of the practice phoneme is achieved.

It is assumed that persons learning the technique have no articulatory deviations. As they practice the manipulations, they should begin by stimulating the target phonemes only. As they become more skilled and are practicing the manipulations on other persons learning the technique, they may wish to practice stimulating the entire syllable or word. Care should be exercised in using materials with respondents. Respondents should not utilize words in which sounds other than the target phoneme are defective.

Chapter 5

PREPARATION AND PLACEMENT OF PHONODENTAL GUIDES

GWENYTH R. VAUGHN, TED A. FULLER, HERNANDO DE CASTRO, JOHNNYE AKIN, AND JAMES S. WALL

- FEDERATION DENTAIRE
- TYPES, PREPARATION, AND PLACEMENT OF PHONODENTAL GUIDES
- Oral Acrylic Modifiers
- Orthodontic Wire Guides
- Denture Guides
- Dental Floss Guides
  - Preparation of Dental Floss Guides
  - Placement of Dental Floss Guides
- Stemmed Wire Guides
  - Preparation of Stemmed Wire Guides
  - Types of Stemmed Wire Guides
- Cue Sticks

FEDERATION DENTAIRE INTERNATIONALE TOOTH NUMBERING SYSTEM

THE FEDERATION DENTAIRE INTERNATIONALE for Designating and Encoding Human Dentition (International Dental Federation Tooth Numbering System) was selected for describing the placement of the phonodental guides. The following outline gives the FDI System and the numbers assigned to the permanent (secondary) teeth. The first digit of the FDI System refers to the *quadrant* of the denture; the second digit indicates the *position* of the tooth from the midline. The Numbering System is illustrated below and in Figures 5 and 6.

Permanent Teeth

(upper right)	(upper left)
18 17 16 15 14 13 12 11	21 22 23 24 25 26 27 28
48 47 46 45 44 43 42 41	31 32 33 34 35 36 37 38
(lower right)	(lower left)

The guides are placed so that the tongue can identify the general articulatory areas for certain sounds. Since the tongue tends to seek contact with foreign objects in the oral cavity, the guides serve as markers for the approximate lingual positions.

The placement of the guides is based on what is generally described as the "ideal" articulation areas for the production of specific phonemes. Small changes in placement make little difference until the articulation boundaries of another sound are crossed. Articulatory compensation, however, often alleviates or compensates for this problem. If it appears that a person responds better to the stimulation from a phonodental guide in a position different from that suggested in the *Manual,* adjustments in the placement of the guides should be made to meet the needs of each respondent. Phonodental guides are *not* intended for use in the *refinement of speech.* They are designed to assist persons with articulation disorders to identify lingual contact areas.

TYPES, PREPARATION, AND PLACEMENT OF PHONODENTAL GUIDES

Phonodental guides consist of (1) oral acrylic modifiers, (2) orthodontic wire guides, (3) denture guides, (4) dental floss guides, (5) stemmed wire guides, and (6) cue sticks. The important contribution of combined intraoral and extraoral stimulations is that intraoral phonodental guides assist in tongue *placement* while extraoral manipulations stimulate *movement* and may serve as a visual aid.

Additional information concerning phonodental guides and cue sticks may be found in Chapter 6 and the Summary in the Appendix.

Oral Acrylic Modifiers

Oral acrylic modifiers for use with dentulous persons were developed by Gwenyth R. Vaughn and James S. Wall in 1967. The design of the modifiers was based on prior investigations of pedodontist Joseph Sim (Sim, 1966; Daniels, Sim, and Simon, 1966).

The oral acrylic modifiers consist of individually-fitted acrylic palates with wire loops placed at points where tongue and alveolar ridge contact are desired. The length of the modifier is adjusted so that it does not interfere with swallowing.

Holes are drilled in the modifier and loops of dental tape are attached. These strands are held in the hands of the stimulator or pinned to the clothes of the respondent so there is no danger of aspiration. Adams Clasps are used in the construction of the modifiers in order to assure proper retention.

The acrylic modifiers are not wholly satisfactory because (1) the construction of the modifiers is time consuming, (2) the taking of the impression is somewhat disagreeable for the respondents, and (3) the use of the modifiers in speech development or speech remediation is questionable because the thickness of the acrylic adds palatal volume.

Orthodontic Wire Guides

In 1967, Hernando de Castro, orthodontist, suggested the use of small "knobs" added to orthodontic bands as a type of intraoral guide. Although orthodontic wires do not break, loosen, or distort lingual and mandibular functions, they are not practical unless the respondent has orthodontic bands already in place. Otherwise, the respondent has to be referred to an orthodontist or other dental specialist for banding.

Denture Guides

The same year that de Castro suggested orthodontic wire guides, denture guides consisting of acrylic "bumps" or imbedded wires were developed by Wall (a dentist) and Vaughn (a speech pathologist) for use with patients wearing full or partial dentures.

The acrylic "bumps" or wires placed in the maxillary denture are only temporary and are removed when they are no longer needed for lingual guidance. The guide wires are curved and imbedded so there is no danger of their becoming loose and aspirated. The guide is of medium-hard stainless steel wire of .020 inch diameter. It is bent into a loop of 3/16 inch inside diameter. It is easily removed by the dentist with no damage to the denture.

ONE DENTURE GUIDE. Raising the tongue is a problem for some respondents, consequently, the placement of one denture guide at the lingua-alveolar contact area above the Maxillary Central Incisors (11-21) usually brings the tongue tip into position for /n, t, d/ (*no*, *to*, *do*). By combining the extraoral manipulations for these sounds with the denture guide, the above phonemes are effectively stimulated. See Figure 5 for placement of the denture guide.

TWO DENTURE GUIDES. Two denture guides may be placed at the lingua-alveolar contact areas above the Maxillary Second Bicuspids and First Molars (15-16 and 25-26). The sides of the tongue usually seek these guides and locate the approximate positions for /ʃ, ʒ/ (*sh*oe, *az*ure), and /i, ɪ, e, ɛ/ (*be*, *it*, v*a*cation, b*e*t). (See Figure 6.)

In approximately the same area, but slightly posterior, /r, j/ (*r*at, *y*et) are located. Between Maxillary First Molars and Second Molars (16-17 and 26-27), approximate contact areas for /ɝ, ɚ/ (b*ir*d, sist*er*), and /u, ʊ, o/ (b*oo*t, f*oo*t, *o*bey) are found. Slightly farther back /k, g, ŋ/ (*k*eep, *g*o, si*ng*) are located. (See Figure 6 for placement of guides.)

The aim of the denture guides is to stimulate the raising of the tongue sides to the approximate alveolar contact areas. The guides may be placed slightly anterior or posterior to the points suggested above depending upon the needs of the respondents. Care should be taken not to place them so far back that the gag reflex is triggered.

Dental Floss Guides

Dental floss guides for use with dentulous persons were developed by Vaughn in 1973. Akin (phonetician) and Wall (dentist) assisted Vaughn in identifying the intraoral placement points for the guides.

Two types of dental floss guides were designed: the knotted guide and the stretched guide.

Preparation of Dental Floss Guides

Most dentists recommend unwaxed dental floss to their patients for home care. The waxed floss, however, is more suitable for fashioning dental floss guides because of its greater body. The unwaxed dental floss, once it is wet, becomes very soft, thus becoming more difficult for the tongue to identify it.

KNOTTED GUIDES. Strands of narrow, waxed dental floss are used. The strand should be long enough for the stimulator to wrap one end firmly around a finger or to make a loop at the same end so it can be pinned to the respondent's clothing. A 15-inch strand usually provides sufficient length for it to be used as either a knotted or stretched guide.

The knot of the knotted guide is tied about 3 inches from the end of the strand. The short extension beyond the knot allows the stimulator to grasp both ends of the strand for easy insertion and removal.

The size of the knot should be adjusted to the interdental spaces of the individual respondent. The knot should be large enough so that it will *not* pull through the space, while the strand is small enough to slip easily between closely spaced teeth. Thicker strands may be chosen for respondents with widely spaced teeth.

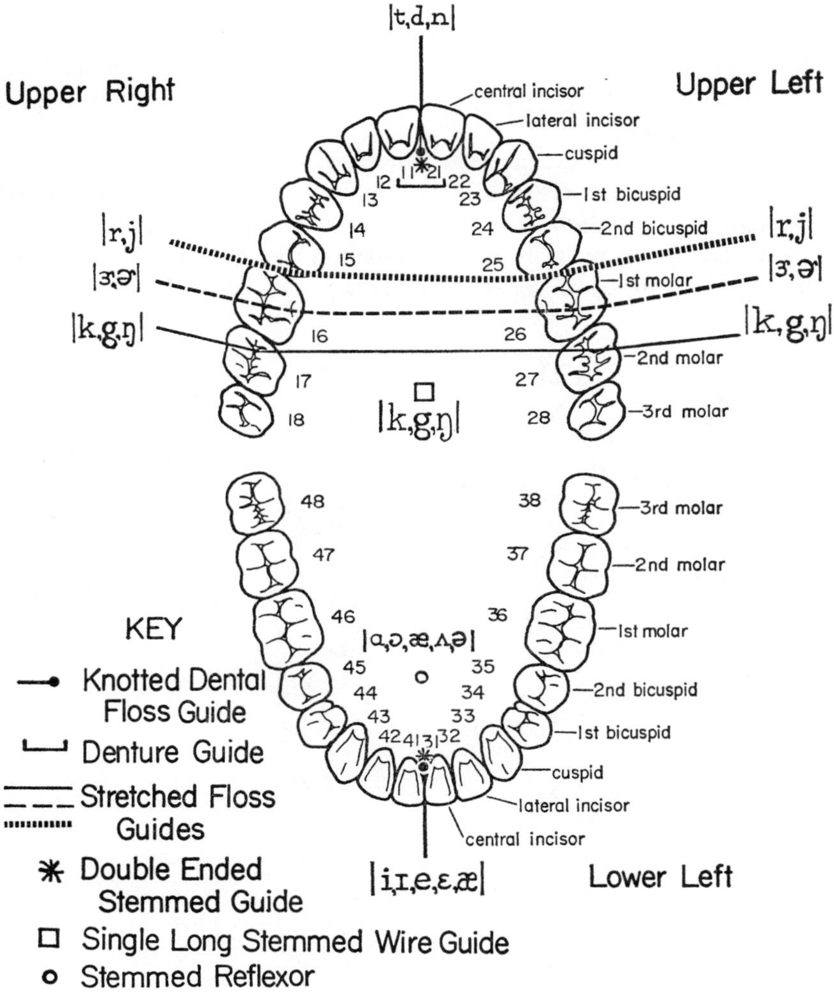

Figure 5. Placement of single and stretched phonodental guides.

Stretched Guide. A single 15-inch strand allows sufficient length for both ends of the strand to be wrapped around a finger of each hand.

Placement of Dental Floss Guides

One Knotted Guide. The placement of the single strand of knotted dental floss guide is related to (1) lifting the tip of the tongue to the alveolar ridge above the Maxillary Central Incisors, and (2) lowering the tip of the tongue to the base of the Mandibular Central Incisors.

The stimulation resulting from the knotted guides is to facilitate lingual placement and should be combined with the extraoral manipulations, whenever necessary, to bring about movement essential to the production and differentiation of the various phonemes. Figure 5 gives the placements.

A single knotted dental floss guide may be placed between the Maxillary Central Incisors (11-21) and combined with appropriate extraoral manipulations to distinguish between frontal and lateral lingua-alveolar contacts for the stimulation of /t, d, n/ (*to*, *do*, *no*) and /l/ (*l*et), for example. (See Figure 5.)

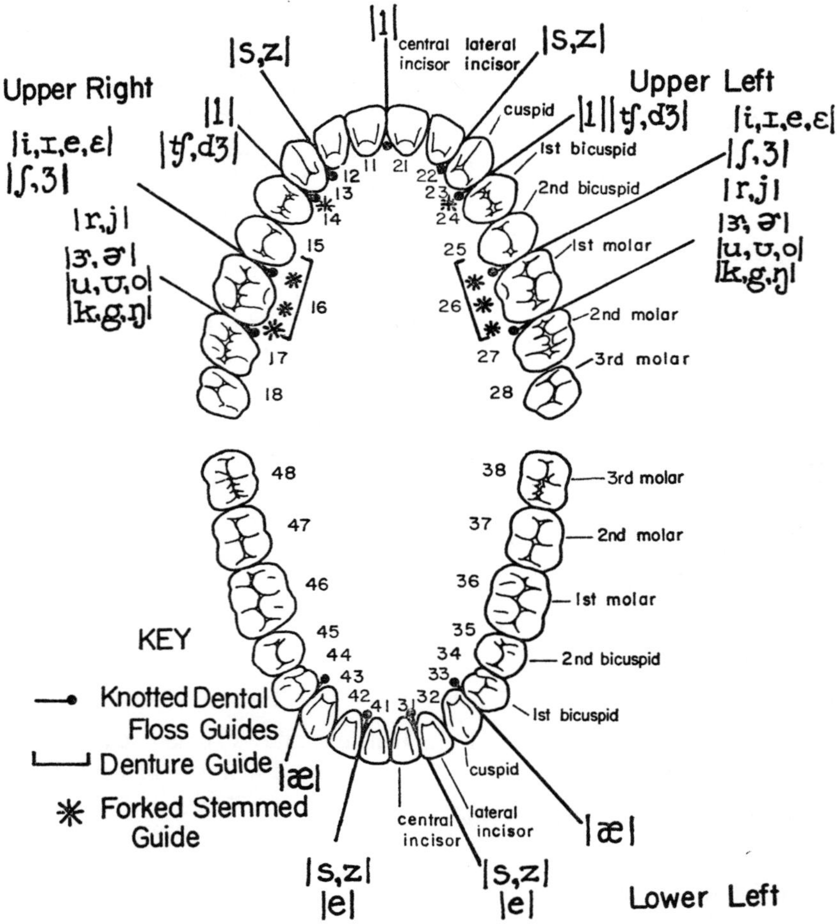

Figure 6. Placement of double phonodental guides.

A single knotted dental guide placed between the Mandibular Central Incisors (31-41) may assist in the production of /i, ɪ, e, ɛ, æ/ (b*e*, *i*t, v*a*cation, b*e*t, *a*t). (See Figure 5.)

Two Knotted Guides. The use of two strands of knotted dental floss may signal the broadening of the tongue tip or the formation of an air channel. See Figure 6 for the placement of two knotted dental guides. The placement of two knotted dental floss guides deep within the oral cavity is often difficult. Stemmed wire guides or cue sticks may be substituted for dental floss guides in the stimulation of these sounds.

Two knotted dental guides placed between Maxillary Lateral Incisors and Cuspids (12-13 and 22-23) may signal /s, z/ (*s*o, *z*one); between Cuspids and First Bicuspids (13-14 and 23-24) may indicate /l, tʃ, dʒ/ (*l*et, *ch*in, *j*am); between Maxillary Second Bicuspids and First Molars (15-16 and 25-26) should encourage the lifting of the tongue for the lingua-alveolar contact for /i, ɪ, e, ɛ/ (b*e*, *i*t, v*a*cation, b*e*t) and /ʃ, ʒ/ (*sh*oe, a*z*ure); and in a slightly posterior position to the latter stimulate /r, j/ (*r*at, *y*et).

Between Maxillary First Molars and Second Molars (16-17 and 26-27), the approximate position for /ɝ, ɚ/ (b*ir*d, sist*er*) and /u, ʊ, o/ (b*oo*t, f*oo*t, *o*bey) may be found. The positions for /r, j/(*r*at, *y*et), /ɝ, ɚ/ (b*ir*d, sist*er*) may be stimulated better by utilizing a stretched dental floss guide.

It is usually too difficult to place two knotted guides between Maxillary First and Second Molars (16-17 and 26-27) for the /k, g, ŋ/ (*k*eep, go, si*ng*). Use of a stretched dental floss guide, a stemmed guide, or cue stick is recommended.

Two knotted dental floss guides may be placed between Mandibular Central and Lateral Incisors (31-32 and 41-42) to signal /e/ (v*a*cation) and /s, z/ (*s*o, *z*one); and between Mandibular Cuspids and Bicuspids (33-34 and 43-44) for /æ/ (*a*t). The sides of the tongue continue to make contact in the areas of the Maxillary Lateral Incisors and Cuspids (12-13 and 22-23) for /s, z/ (*s*o, *z*one), even if the tongue tip is lowered. The /s, z/ (*s*o, *z*one) mandibular tongue tip placements are alternate placements for the Maxillary contact areas. Stimulation with the short prong of the stemmed reflexor or a cue stick may be used.

Three Knotted Guides. Three knotted dental floss guides placed at the lingua-alveolar contact areas above the Maxillary Central Incisors (11-21) and between the Maxillary Cuspids and First Bicuspids (13-14 and 23-24) stimulate /l/ (*l*et). (See Figure 6.)

STRETCHED GUIDE. The stretched guides may be placed across the crowns of the maxillary teeth to encourage the lifting of the tongue. As the tongue makes contact with the strand, the dental floss can be relaxed so the tongue assumes a broader contact with the palate. The extraoral manipulations can then be used to indicate the movement of the tongue in the areas of the Maxillary Second Bicuspids and First Molars (15-16 and 25-26) or at the First Molars (15-16 and 25-26) or at the First Molars (16-26) for /r, j/ (*r*at, *y*et); and in the area of the Maxillary First Molars (16 and 26) or slightly posterior for /ɝ, ɚ/ (b*ir*d, sist*er*); and in the approximate area of Maxillary Second Molars (17 and 27) for /k, g, ŋ/ (*k*eep, *g*o, si*ng*). Figure 5 gives the approximate placements.

Stemmed Wire Guides

In 1976, Ted A. Fuller, speech pathologist and educator of the deaf, suggested the use of stemmed wire guides as an approach to improved tongue placement. Hernando de Castro, an orthodontist, designed, in cooperation with Fuller and Vaughn, the first sets of stemmed wire guides. These are used singly or in combination with the extraoral manipulations. They consist of wire with curved ends to provide safe surfaces for stimulating specific points in the oral cavity while permitting a secure handhold at the other end. The wire stems are slender and thus do not interfere with tongue movement.

The stimulator holds a dental mirror in one hand so the desired contact point in the oral cavity is reflected while the stemmed wire guide is placed and/or held in place by the other hand. If the mirror tends to steam, it may be dipped in warm water. After the guide is in place, the dental mirror is put aside, freeing that hand for application of the extraoral manipulations.

Preparation of Stemmed Wire Guides

The use of standard segments of medium-hard stainless steel wire facilitates the construction of the stemmed wire guides. This wire may be purchased from dental supply houses. Only one segment, or a part of one segment, is needed for each guide.

Pliers used in bending the wires may be purchased from dental supply houses or local hardware stores. The pliers are designated as bird beak pliers with one short round beak and one square beak.

Figures 7 and 8 illustrate the various types of stemmed wire guides. The drawings are full size, and the guides may be constructed by placing the wires over the illustrations and bending the wires to con-

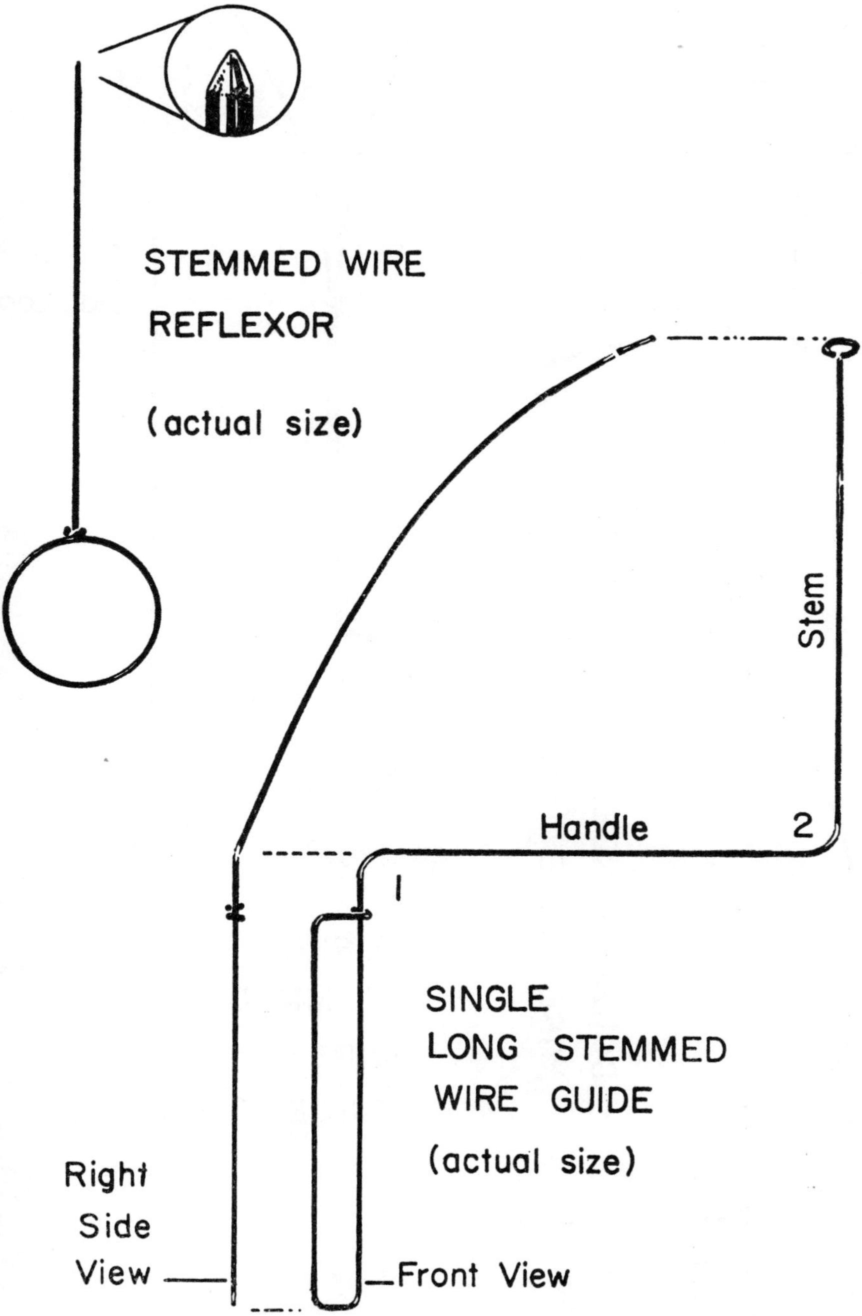

Figure 7. Stemmed wire reflexor and single long stemmed wire guide.

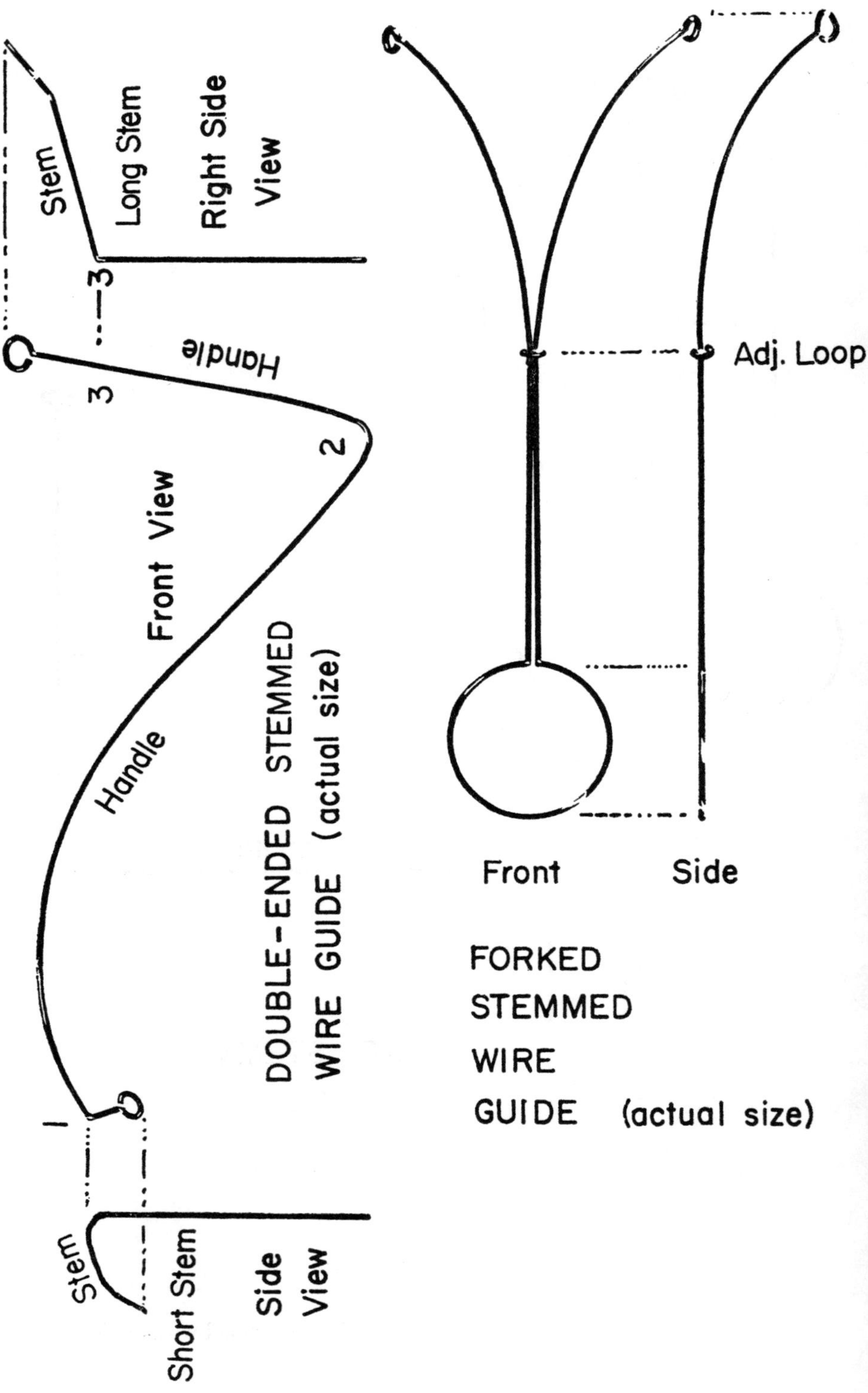

Figure 8. Double-ended stemmed wire guide and forked stemmed wire guide.

form with the lines in the figures and the descriptions offered in the following paragraphs.

Types of Stemmed Wire Guides

Four types of stemmed wire guides are utilized: (1) stemmed wire reflexor, (2) double-ended stemmed wire guide, (3) single long stemmed wire guide, and (4) forked stemmed wire guide. Figures 7 and 8 illustrate the stemmed wire guides. The handles of these guides have been designed so they do not interfere with the hand that is applying the extraoral manipulations.

STEMMED WIRE REFLEXOR. The stemmed wire reflexor is constructed of medium-hard stainless steel wire of .028 inch in diameter. One end is pointed; the other end has a wire circle to accommodate the index finger of the stimulator. The circle should be slipped beyond the first knuckle in order to provide a firm grasp between the finger and thumb.

This reflexor is made from a piece of wire 4½ inches long. The handle consists of a circle of about ¾ inches in diameter; the stem is 2½ inches long. The end has a conical point made by filing, or by using a polishing stone or a carborundum disc. (See Figure 7.)

The reflexor is used to lower the tongue. Extraoral manipulations assist in positioning the mandible and indicating the degree of lip rounding for the phonemes /ɑ, æ, ɔ, ʌ, ə/ (c*a*lm and l*o*t; *a*t; w*ar* and s*aw*; c*u*p, sof*a*). The stemmed reflexor is also used to position the tongue for the first elements of the diphthong /ɑi, ɔi, ɔu/ (m*i*ce, b*oy*, c*ow*), the extraoral manipulations define the first element and then move the lips into position for the second element.

The rationale for using the stemmed wire reflexor is that the sharp point causes the tongue to assume a low position in the mouth. If the respondent only retracts the tip of the tongue, the stimulator may touch the dorsum of the tongue in order to stimulate the retraction of the body of the tongue. A tongue depressor is often utilized to push the tongue into a low position. The tongue, however, tends to pull back instead of assuming the desired position.

DOUBLE-ENDED STEMMED WIRE GUIDE. The double-ended stemmed wire guide is constructed of medium-hard stainless steel wire of .028 inches in diameter. For better oral placement, the stems at each end are different lengths. The shorter stem is used for mandibular stimulation and the longer stem for maxillary stimulation. The handle is bent into a right angle, thus permitting the stimulator to grasp it easily, regardless of whether the long or short stem is being utilized.

This double-ended stemmed guide is made of a piece of wire

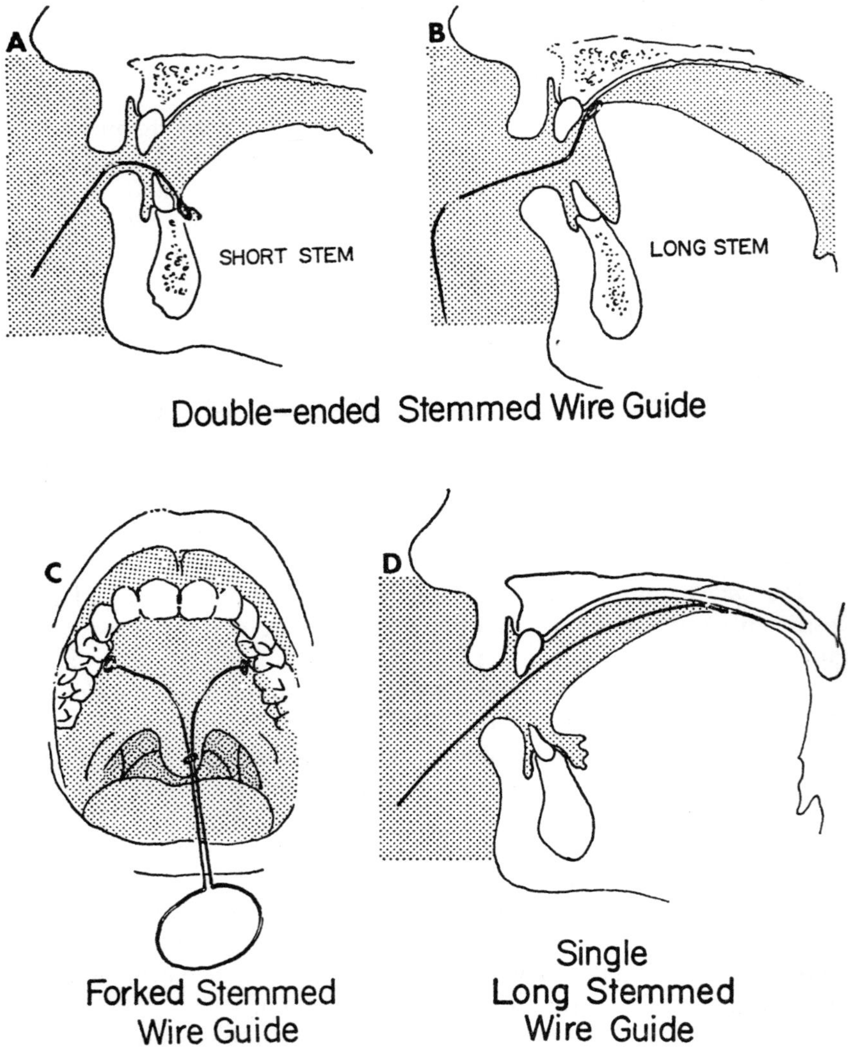

Figure 9. Placement of stemmed wire guides.

9-10 inches long. The handle consists of a section of wire that is 7½ inches from bend 1 through bend 2 and up to bend 3. The shorter stem is ⅝ inch long; the longer stem is 1¼ inches in length. The circles at the ends of the stems are of ⅛ inch inside diameter. (See Figure 8.)

The stems are placed at a 90° angle to the handles. To complete the additional curvature of the stems after the 90° angle, see Figure 8. It is suggested that the wire be placed over the front view in the illustration in order to achieve the handle curvature and make 90° bends at points 1 and 3. In order to prepare the long stem, the end of the wires should be superimposed upon the right side view; the same procedure should be followed by superimposing the other end of the wire upon the left side view.

The circles of ⅛ inch inside diameter at the ends of both stems should then be completed.

The circle at the end of the longer stem is placed on the lingual side of the alveolar ridge at the point above and between Maxillary Central Incisors (11-21) in order to stimulate the /t, d, n/ (*to*, *do*, *no*). The guide is removed after the tongue has assumed its place or, if extraoral manipulations are combined with the guide, it is removed simultaneously with the flick of the index finger. (See Figure 9-B.)

The circle at the end of the shorter stem may be used to position the tongue tip behind the Mandibular Central Incisors (31-41) for /i, ɪ, e, ɜ, æ/ (b*e*, *i*t, v*a*cation, b*e*t, *a*t). It may also be used to stroke the mid-line of the tip of the tongue to encourage grooving for /ɪ/ (*i*t). See Figures 5 and 9-A. The shorter stem may also be used for sounds stimulated from this basic position and differentiated by extraoral manipulations. These sounds include /e, æ/ (v*a*cation, *a*t) and /s, z/ (*s*o, *z*one). (See Figures 6 and 9-A.)

Single Long-stemmed Wire Guide. The single long-stemmed wire guide is constructed of medium-hard stainless steel wire of .028 inch in diameter. The guide is made from a piece of wire 11 inches long. The handle consists of a rectangular loop of wire 2″ × ¼″. (See Figure 7.) Curve 1 is at a 90° angle; curve 2 is also 90°. The stem from the curve to the circular tip is 3⅜ inches long. The curvature complies with the right side view. The circle at the tip is ⅛ inch inside diameter.

This single long stemmed wire guide is used to touch the velum at the point at which the linguavelar contact produces the /k, g, ŋ/ (*k*eep, *g*o, si*ng*). The guide is removed after the tongue has assumed its place or, if extraoral manipulations are combined with the guide, it is removed simultaneously with the release of manipulation. (See Figure 9-D.)

The single long stemmed wire guide may be used to raise the tongue or to indicate maxillary contact areas.

Forked Stemmed Wire Guide. The forked stemmed wire guide is constructed of medium-hard stainless steel wire of .028 inch in diameter. The guide is made from a piece of wire and is 11 to 12 inches long.

The handle consists of a circle of ¾ inch diameter; the stems are each 4 inches long. At 2 inches from the circular handle, the stems diverge into compound curves that terminate in small circles of ⅛ inch inside diameter. An adjustment loop no longer than ⅛ inch outside diameter is constructed and clasped around the two stems. This loop controls the spread of the circular tips by sliding up and down the stems.

To make this forked stemmed wire guide, (1) establish mid-point of wire, (2) form a ¾ inch diameter circle at the mid-point, (3) bend the stems according to the diagram, following both the front and side views, (4) at 4 inches from the circular handle, complete the circles of ⅛ inch inside diameter.

The forked stemmed wire guide has a circle to accommodate the index finger just above the knuckle. (See Figure 8.)

By placing the tips of the prongs on the lingual side of the lateral maxillary alveolar ridges in the approximate areas of the Maxillary Cuspids and first Bicuspids (13-14 and 23-24), the /l, tʃ, dʒ/ (*l*et, *ch*in, *j*am) may be stimulated; between the Maxillary Second Bicuspids and First Molars (15-16 and 25-26), the /i, ɪ, e, æ/ (b*e*, *i*t, v*a*cation, *a*t) and /ʃ, ʒ/ (*sh*oe, a*z*ure); in a slightly posterior position, the /r, j/ (*r*at, *y*et) may be located; at approximately the Maxillary First Molars (16 and 26), the /ɝ, ɚ/ (b*ir*d, sist*er*); and between the Maxillary First Molars and Second Molars (16-17 and 26-27), the /u, ʊ, o/ (b*oo*t, f*oo*t, *o*bey) and /k, g, ŋ/ (*k*eep, *g*o, si*ng*) can be stimulated.

The guide is removed after the tongue has assumed its place. If extraoral manipulations are combined with the guide, it is removed simultaneously with the release of finger pressure. Mandibular closure and lip extension determine the specific phoneme.

The most important use of the forked stemmed wire guide is for positioning the tongue for the /r, j/ (*r*at, *y*et) and /ɝ, ɚ/ (b*ir*d, sist*er*). The tip of the tongue is engaged by the fork so that the tongue body is pushed back and up to the approximate positions described in the preceding paragraph. (See Figures 6 and 9-C.)

The placement of the forked stemmed wire guide is adjusted to what appears to be the optimal contact area of the individual respondents. The guide is removed after the tongue has assumed its place or, if extraoral manipulations are combined with the guide, it is removed simultaneously with the release of the manipulation.

Cue Sticks

Cue sticks consist of cotton-tipped sticks dipped in cold water and tongue depressors. The cotton-tipped sticks and the tongue depressors are placed at the same points suggested for the other phonodental guides.

COTTON-TIPPED GUIDES. Cotton-tipped guides such as Q-Tips® are dipped in cold water in order to heighten the intraoral sensation. The cotton is firmly wrapped so that no danger of aspiration exists.

TONGUE DEPRESSORS. Tongue depressors may be broken into narrow lengths, if desired.

Note: The Appendix provides a master chart that summarizes the movements of the extraoral manipulations and the placements of the phonodental guides for each phoneme.

SECTION III

SPEECH FACILITATION MANUAL

INTRODUCTION

SPEECH FACILITATION stimulations help the respondent feel, as well as hear and see speech. The technique helps the respondent establish effective positions and movements essential to the production of speech sounds. The stimulations also contribute to the respondent's understanding of the articulation patterns characteristic of each phoneme.

In the Speech Facilitation approach to the production of speech sounds, the interest is not in delicate refinement of sounds but rather in broad concepts and basic communication.

Section III Organization

Chapter 6 includes the Stimulation Units for specific phonemes. It is divided into Sections devoted to groups of vowels, diphthongs, and consonants. The Stimulation Units are self-contained and may be taught in any order. Practice materials are provided for each Unit; comparative practice materials are included at the end of each Section.

Chapter 7 discusses the suggested practice order. Sounds are most easily taught by the Speech Facilitation technique when extreme vowels are combined with the consonants. Practice materials are also included for each group of phonemes based on this order.

The Appendix provides a master chart that summarizes the extraoral manipulations and intraoral placements of phonodental guides.

Chapter 6

STIMULATION SECTIONS AND UNITS

- SECTIONS FOR VOWELS AND DIPHTHONGS
- Section A: Front Vowels (Stimulation Units 1-4)
- Section B: Back Vowels (Stimulation Units 5-8)
- Section C: Central Vowels (Stimulation Units 9-10)
- Section D: Diphthongs (Stimulation Units 11-16)
- SECTIONS FOR CONSONANTS
- Section E: Nasal Continuants (Stimulation Units 17-19)
- Section F: Stop Plosives (Stimulation Units 20-22)
- Section G: Fricatives (Part 1) (Stimulation Units 23-25)
- Section H: Fricatives and Affricates (Part 2) (Stimulation Units 26-28)
- Section I: Fricatives and Semivowels (Stimulation Units 29-32)

Overview of Stimulation Unit

Each Stimulation Unit contains the following information:

STIMULATION UNIT NUMBER
Phonetic Symbol and Representative Word
Symbol Systems
Topographical Relationships of Phoneme Production
Stimulation Procedures
Extraoral Manipulation
Response Analysis and Extraoral Cues
Phonodental Guides
Selected Phoneme Characteristics
Practice Materials

Additional information related to the extraoral manipulations may be found in Chapter 4 and the Appendix. Further details regarding the phonodental guides are located in Chapter 5 and the Appendix.

References for the background material on symbol systems and selected phoneme characteristics follow:

Symbol Systems

The symbol systems include the International Phonetic Alphabet, *Webster's New Collegiate Dictionary* (1965), *Thorndike-Barnhardt Comprehensive Dictionary* (1951), and Northampton Charts (Yale, 1946).

Selected Phoneme Characteristics

DEVELOPMENTAL AGE. The developmental age as given by Templin (1957) provides a baseline for the chronological age at which articulation skills may be considered within normal limits.

FREQUENCY OF OCCURRENCE OF PHONEME. The occurrence of each phoneme is expressed in relative percentages and in order of occurrence according to Hutton (1969).

VISUAL INTELLIGIBILITY. The range of intelligibility is provided as well as the composite percentage of several studies from Heider and Heider (1940), Samuelson (1943), O'Neill (1954), Hutton (1959), Woodward (1957), and Hutton (1969).

VISUAL CONFUSION. Hutton (1969) prepared a chart of visual confusion from which the visual confusion characteristics are taken.

AUDITORY INTELLIGIBILITY. The percentage of auditory intelligibility of each phoneme for persons with mild-to-severe hearing impairments is given (Hutton, 1959).

AUDITORY CONFUSION. Hutton (1969) developed a chart for the phonemes in which auditory confusion is likely to take place. The auditory confusion characteristics are taken from the Hutton chart.

RELATIVE PHONETIC POWER. The relative phonetic power of each sound is taken from Fletcher (1953).

PHONEMIC CONFUSION. Van Riper and Irwin (1958) prepared diagrams that displayed the phonemes that are most likely to be confused. Information from these diagrams is given.

TYPICAL SPELLING. Sample words are taken from several sources easily available to most clinicians and are used to illustrate the various ways of representing a certain sound.

Practice Materials

All examples of pronunciations used in this book in the parts on Typical Spelling and Practice Materials are standard pronunciations.

Individual pronunciations may vary from area to area; if regional differences are apparent, an acceptable pronunciation to the specific region should be used for practice.

Practice materials are placed at the end of each Stimulation Unit. Comparative practice materials for trainees and for selective use with respondents may be found at the end of each Section in Chapter 6 and after each group of phonemes in Chapter 7. It is assumed that the trainees have no articulatory deviations. At first, only the target phonemes in the practice words should be stimulated. When satisfactory facilitation in the use of the technique is achieved, trainees may practice stimulating a complete word in order to develop greater skill.

Although trainees will probably first learn the stimulations for the sounds in the initial position, some respondents may first learn the sound better in the final position.

Care should be exercised in using these materials with respondents. Words including sounds that are defective—other than the target phoneme—should not be utilized with respondents.

Evaluation

Each clinician should use an evaluation instrument that will provide a baseline as well as interim and post-treatment scores.

Sections for Vowels and Diphthongs

Introduction

The Sections consist of front vowels, back vowels, central vowels, and diphthongs. The front and back vowels are further divided into high, medial, and low vowels. The low front intermediate IPA Symbol /a/ and the low back tense vowel IPA symbol /ɒ/ have been omitted because they are identified with regional pronunciation, and it is not necessary to discuss the intricacies involved in their production and use. Figure 10 gives the approximate topographical location for the vowels and diphthongs.

In the Speech Facilitation approach to the production of speech sounds, the interest is not in delicate refinement of sounds but rather in broad concepts and basic communication. The diphthongs illustrate this principle: it is easier to stimulate /ɑu/ (*cow*) than /aʊ/ (*cow*). The latter sound adjustment takes place as it becomes assimilated into fast, facile speech patterns, and the diphthong seems to take the form of /aʊ/. Both are acceptable pronunciations.

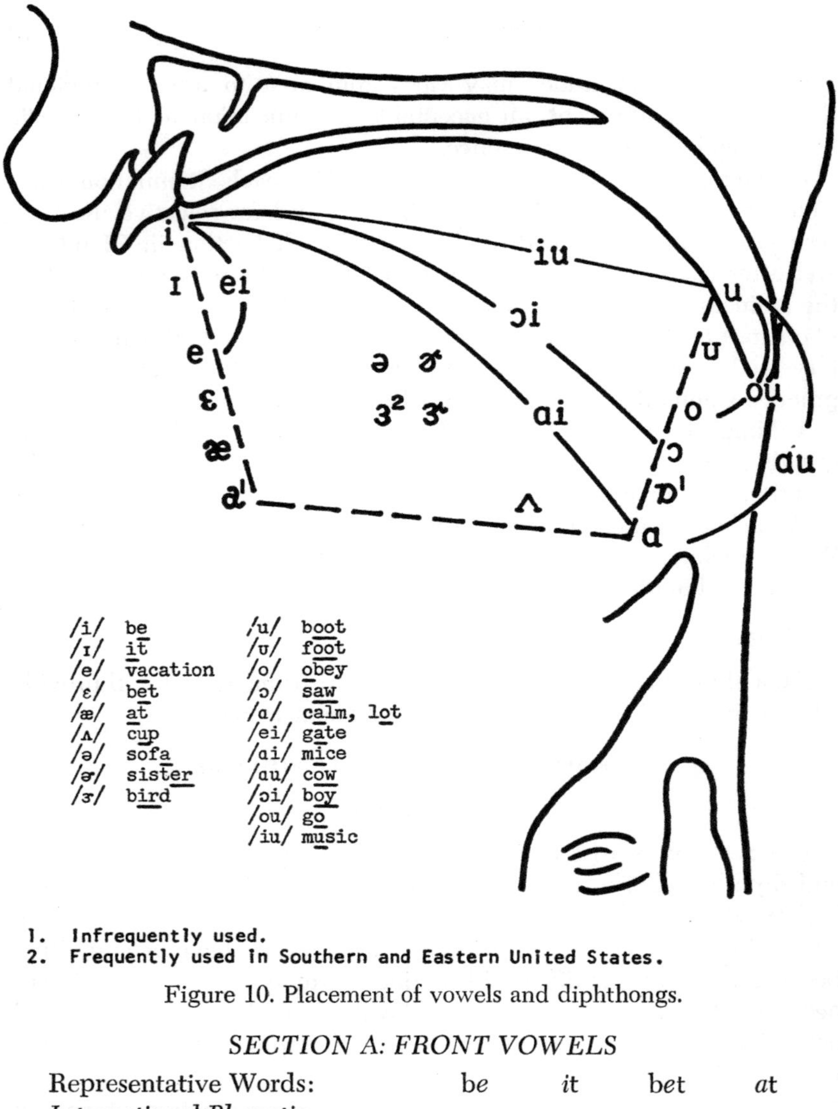

1. Infrequently used.
2. Frequently used in Southern and Eastern United States.

Figure 10. Placement of vowels and diphthongs.

SECTION A: FRONT VOWELS

Representative Words:	b*e*	*i*t	b*e*t	*a*t
International Phonetic Alphabet:	/i/	/ɪ/	/ɛ/	/æ/
Webster's New Collegiate Dictionary (1965):	ē	ĭ	ĕ	ă
Thorndike-Barnhardt Comprehensive Dictionary (1951):	ē	i	e, ã	a
Northampton Charts (Yale, 1946):	ee	-i-	-e-	-a-

Stimulation Units are provided for the four front vowels. These include the high front, tense, unrounded /i/ (b*e*), high front, lax, unrounded /ɪ/ (*i*t), mid front, lax, unrounded /ɛ/ (b*e*t), and low front, tense, unrounded /æ/ (*a*t). The mid front, tense, unrounded /e/ (v*a*cation) is discussed under the diphthong /ei/ (g*a*te) in Stimulation Unit 12.

All of the front vowels have certain characteristics in common insofar as production is concerned. The two important factors concerned with the production of the front vowels are the position of the tongue and the depression of the mandible to the lowest unstrained position. For all of these sounds /i/ (b*e*), /ɪ/ (*i*t), /ɛ/ (b*e*t), and /æ/ (*a*t), the apex of the tongue is posterior to the lingual surface of the mandibular incisors and remains in this position for all of the front vowel sounds. The body of the tongue is arched anteriorly to the primary palate. As the mandible is progressively depressed, the tongue follows the depression and gradually flattens as it loses contact with the upper teeth.

Between the mid and low front sounds /ɛ/ (b*e*t) and /æ/ (*a*t), there is approximately 5 to 7 mm depression, and it is at this point that the tongue loses all contact with the upper teeth. If the tongue remains in contact with the upper teeth during the production of the /æ/ (*a*t) sound, it usually results in nasality, which causes a distortion of quality.

Stimulation Unit 1

Phonetic Symbol and Representative Word: /i/ (b*e*)

Symbol Systems

International Phonetic Alphabet: /i/
Webster's New Collegiate Dictionary (1965): ē
Thorndike-Barnhardt Comprehensive Dictionary (1951): ē
Northampton Charts (Yale, 1946): ee

Topographical Relationships of Phoneme Production
/i/ (b*e*) high front tense unrounded

MANDIBLE:
slightly lowered from position of closure

LIPS:
drawn back in tense position; opening appears as long horizontal line

TONGUE:

Tip—at or near base of lower front teeth

Body—arched and forward

Sides—in contact with maxillary molars

AIRSTREAM:

emitted through small forward opening between tongue and palate

NASAL PORT:

closed

VOCAL FOLDS:

vibrating

Stimulation Procedures

VISUAL-AUDITORY MODEL. A model demonstration is provided by the manipulation of the stimulator's face while the respondent observes. An auditory stimulus is usually given simultaneously as the stimulator is saying: "We are going to say /i/ (b*e*)." This step may be repeated.

STARTING POSITION. Respondent's articulators should be in the starting position before the manipulation is initiated: lips parted; mandible lowered slightly from position of closure; tongue in customary, relaxed position; vocal folds not vibrating.

SIMULTANEOUS STIMULATION. Stimulator places fingers in position on respondent's face. As the manipulation takes place, the respondent may observe the stimulator's face and/or hear an auditory stimulus.

EXTRAORAL MANIPULATION /i/ (b*e*)

1. Assume starting position.
2. Place thumb and middle finger of one hand on upper lip points 2.
3. Press inward and slide fingers simultaneously toward upper lip points 3—stretching lips into "smile position."
4. Phonate.

If the above manipulation is not sufficient, use the additional manipulation procedures.

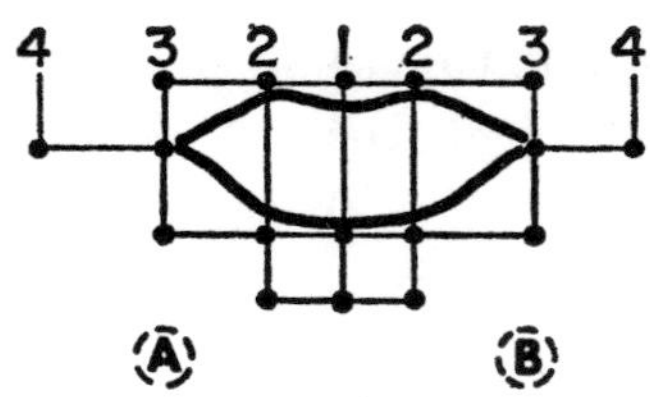

MANIPULATION MODEL: LIPS FORMAT.

ADDITIONAL MANIPULATION

1. Return to starting position.
2. Place thumb and middle finger of one hand on upper lip points 2.
3. Place thumb and middle finger of other hand on lower lip points 2.
4. Press inward and slide finger of both hands simultaneously toward side points 3—stretching lips into "smile position."
5. Phonate. (The stimulator may signal phonation by placing little finger against respondent's larynx.)

/i/ (b*e*) Response Analysis and Extraoral Cues

MANDIBLE. If there is a tendency for the mandible to be lowered more than is appropriate for the /i/(b*e*) sound, the little finger of the hand used to stimulate the lower lip may be hooked under the chin to prevent excessive mandibular depression. Moving the mandible gently up and down can generally bring about greater relaxation of the mandible and other articulators.

LIPS. Lips are usually not rounded on the front vowels. The stimulation and positioning of the lips for the /i/ (b*e*) sound should be conducted with equal pressure and timing on both sides of the mid-line. If the respondent's lips are too tense, the stimulator should gently assist the respondent in moving the lips from a puckered position to the stretched position. The motion should be repeated until the lips are relaxed.

TEETH. In producing the /i/ (b*e*) sound, the teeth are nearly in occlusion. Some persons need to have teeth in occlusion during the first few practice sessions, in order to produce the /i/ (b*e*) sound. Even in this position, however, teeth should not be clinched. This latter position does not interfere with the manipulation of the lips as described above.

TONGUE. The sides of the tongue press against the upper molars. The pressure of the thumb and finger sliding from upper lip points 2 to 3 usually brings the sides of the tongue in contact with the alveolar ridge.

NASAL PORT. If the airstream is being emitted through the nose, the stimulator can place the index finger under the nose of the respondent in order to indicate that the airstream is being improperly emitted. The stimulator should accompany the *tactile* cue with the visual cue of shaking his head "no" or an *auditory* cue by saying "no."

VOCAL FOLDS. The stimulator's little finger may be placed against the respondent's larynx to signal phonation.

/i/ (b*e*) PHONODENTAL GUIDES

Chapter 5 gives details concerning preparation and placement of phonodental guides. Figures 5 and 6 in Chapter 5 illustrate the approximate points of lingual contact for the guides.

Phonodental guides and intraoral cues may be used independently or in combination with the extraoral manipulations.

The extraoral manipulation is usually effective for eliciting this phoneme, and intraoral stimulation is not required. If intraoral stimulation is needed, one or more of the following phonodental guides may be utilized.

Denture Guides /i/ (be)

Denture guides are not usually utilized for identifying points of lingual contact, unless other sounds are involved. (See Figure 6.)

Dental Floss Guides /i/ (be)

Lower tongue tip: one knotted dental-floss guide placed between Mandibular Central Incisors (31-41).

Raised tongue sides: two knotted dental floss guides placed between Maxillary Second Bicuspids and First Molars (15-16 and 25-26).

Stemmed Wire Guides /i/ (be)

Lower tongue tip: shorter stem of double-ended wire guide used to position tongue tip behind Mandibular Central Incisors (31-41).

Raise tongue sides: tips of forked stemmed wire guide adjusted so tips touch aveolar ridge in approximate area of Maxillary Second Bicuspids and First Molars (15-16 and 25-26).

Cue Sticks /i/ (be)

Cotton-tipped sticks dipped in cold water or parts of tongue depressors may be used to stimulate the same points for lingual contact as those given above.

Note: This sound is easily stimulated and is one of the basic vowels used in syllables and words for stimulating target consonant sounds.

/i/ (be) SELECTED PHONEME CHARACTERISTICS

DEVELOPMENTAL AGE:[1]

3 years

FREQUENCY OF OCCURRENCE OF PHONEME:[2]

1.82%; twenty-second in order of occurrence

VISUAL INTELLIGIBILITY:[3]

range—33% to 77%; composite 58%

VISUAL CONFUSION:[4]

not given

AUDITORY INTELLIGIBILITY IN MILD-TO-SEVERE HEARING IMPAIRMENTS:[5]
80%

AUDITORY CONFUSION:[6]
/i, ɪ/ (b*e*, *i*t)

RELATIVE PHONETIC POWER:[7]
220 (range of 1 to 680)

PHONEMIC CONFUSION:[8]
/i/ (b*e*); /j/ (*y*et); /ɪ/ (*i*t); /e/ (v*a*cation)

TYPICAL SPELLING:
ae (C*ae*sar); *e* (m*e*); *ee* (n*ee*d); *ea* (*ea*t); *eo* (p*eo*ple); *ey* (k*ey*; *ei* (rec*ei*pt); *ie* (f*ie*ld); *i* (mach*i*ne); *oe* (ph*oe*nix); *uay* (q*uay*)

/i/ (b*e*)PRACTICE MATERIALS

The sound to be stimulated is /i/ (b*e*). Only those words and phrases in which the respondent can articulate all of the sounds correctly, except for the target phoneme, should be utilized for practice. The same stipulation applies to the comparative practice materials provided at the end of this Section.

/h/ he, heap, heat, he's; /p/ pea, peep, peak, Pete; /b/ be, bean, beet, bees; /t/ eat, tea, team, teeth; /d/ Eden, Dee, deep, idea; /k/ eke, key, keen, keep; /g/ ego, Aggie, geese, ghee; /m/ emit, me, meat, meal; /n/ Enid, knee, neat, need; /hw/ whee, wheat, wheel, wheeze; /w/ we, weep, weak, weed; /f/ fee, feet, feed, feel; /v/ eve, even, Vea, veal; /θ/ ether, three, theme; /ð/ either, the, these; /s/ east, see, seen, seat; /z/ ease, easy, Zeke, zeal; /ʃ/ she, sheep, sheet, machine; /ʒ/ Bijou; /tʃ/ each, cheap, cheek, chief; /dʒ/ Egypt, gee, Jean, jeep; /l/ ell, Lee, leap, leaf; /r/ Rhee, ream, read, receive; /j/ ye, yield. *Phrases:* We see Edie. Keith keeps bees. Pete eats meat.

Stimulation Unit 2

Phonetic Symbol and Representative Word: /ɪ/ (*i*t)

Symbol Systems

International Phonetic Alphabet: /ɪ/
Webster's New Collegiate Dictionary (1965): ĭ
Thorndike-Barnhardt Comprehensive Dictionary (1951): i
Northampton Charts (Yale, 1946): -i-

[1] Templin, 1957, p. 51; [2] Tobias, 1959, p. 631; [3] Hutton, 1969, p. 113; [4] Hutton, 1969, p. 114; [5] Hutton, 1959, pp. 319-329; [6] Hutton, 1969, p. 128; [7] Fletcher, 1953, p. 86; [8] Van Riper and Irwin, 1958, p. 72. Hereafter, the references will be listed in the foregoing order.

Topographical Relationships of Phoneme Production
/ɪ/ (*i*t) high front lax unrounded

MANDIBLE:
slightly lower than for /i/ (b*e*)

LIPS:
less everted than for /i/ (b*e*) and with corners slightly inward

TONGUE:
Tip—at or near base of lower front teeth
Body—begins to drop from high, tense position of /i/
Sides—in contact with maxillary molars

AIRSTREAM:
emitted through small opening between tongue and hard palate

NASAL PORT:
closed

VOCAL FOLDS:
vibrating

Stimulation Procedures

VISUAL-AUDITORY MODEL. A model demonstration is provided by the manipulation of the stimulator's face while the respondent observes. An auditory stimulus is usually given simultaneously as the stimulator is saying: "We are going to say /ɪ/ (*i*t)." This step may be repeated.

STARTING POSITION. Respondent's articulators should be in the starting position before the manipulation is initiated: lips parted; mandible lowered slightly from position of closure; tongue in customary, relaxed position; vocal folds not vibrating.

SIMULTANEOUS STIMULATION. Stimulator places fingers in position on respondent's face. As the manipulation takes place, the respondent may observe the stimulator's face and/or hear an auditory stimulus.

EXTRAORAL MANIPULATION /ɪ/ (*i*t)

1. Assume starting position.
2. Place side of index finger on lower lip point 1.
3. Use tip of index finger; draw a line between lower lip points 1 and mid-chin point 1. (This stimulation should be repeated until the desired sound emerges.)
4. Phonate.

If the above manipulation is not sufficient, use the additional manipulation procedures.

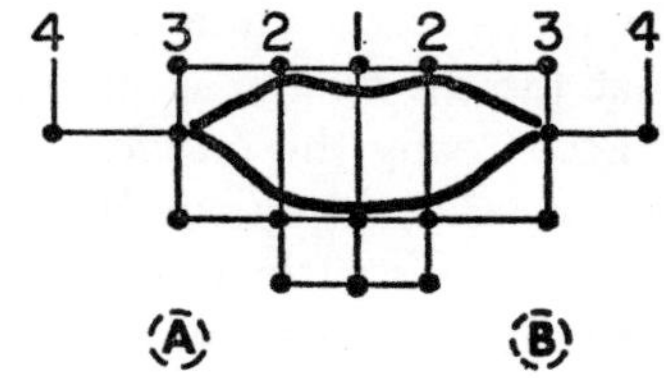

MANIPULATION MODEL: LIPS FORMAT.

ADDITIONAL MANIPULATION

If light stimulation does not produce sound, exert greater pressure with the tip of the index finger in a line between lower lip point 1 and mid-chin point 1. By applying the principle of phonetic derivation, an /ɪ/ (*i*t) can be derived from /i/ (b*e*) by initiating the /i/ (b*e*) first and blending into the /ɪ/ (*i*t) sound. The tongue should dip in response to the stimulation.

1. Return to starting position.
2. Place thumb and middle finger of one hand on lower lip points 2. (Stimulation for /i/ (b*e*).)
3. Press inward and slide fingers simultaneously toward mid-lip points 3—stretching lips into "smile position."
4. Phonate. (Remove upper fingers; begin /ɪ/ (*i*t) manipulation.)
5. Place side of index finger on lower lip point 1.
6. Use tip of index finger to draw a line between lower lip point 1 and mid-chin point 1. (This stimulation should be repeated until the desired sound emerges.)
7. Phonation will have been initiated for /i/ (b*e*) and will continue as the /ɪ/ (*i*t) sound is derived from the first phoneme. (The stimulator may signal phonation by placing little finger against respondent's larynx.)

/ɪ/ (*i*t) Response Analysis and Extraoral Cues

MANDIBLE. If there is a tendency for the mandible to be lowered more than is appropriate for the /ɪ/ (*i*t) sound, the little finger of the hand used to stimulate lower lip may be hooked under the chin to prevent excessive mandibular depression.

LIPS. The lips are lax and unrounded. If the lips are too tense, a gentle shaking movement of the lower lip may help relaxation.

TONGUE. The manipulation is designed to bring a dip along the lingual mid-line at the tongue tip. The vertical enlargement between the arch of the palate and the groove of the tongue is greater than in the /i/ (b*e*) sound.

NASAL PORT. If the airstream is being emitted through the nose, the stimulator can place the index finger under the nose of the respondent in order to indicate that the air stream is being improperly emitted. The stimulator should accompany the *tactile* cue with the *visual* cue of shaking his head "no" or an *auditory* cue by saying "no."

VOCAL FOLDS. The stimulator's little finger may be placed against the respondent's larynx to signal phonation.

/ɪ/ (*i*t) PHONODENTAL GUIDES

Chapter 5 gives details concerning preparation and placement of phonodental guides. Figures 5 and 6 in Chapter 5 illustrate the approximate points of lingual contact for the guides.

Phonodental guides and intraoral cues may be used independently or in combination with the extraoral manipulations. If intraoral stimulation is needed, one or more of the following phonodental guides may be utilized.

Denture Guides /ɪ/ (*i*t)

Denture guides are not usually utilized for identifying points of lingual contact, unless other sounds are involved. (see Figure 6.)

Dental Floss Guides /ɪ/ (*i*t)

Lower tongue tip: one knotted dental floss guide placed between Mandibular Central Incisors (31-41).

Raise tongue sides: two knotted dental floss guides placed between Maxillary Second Bicuspids and First Molars (15-16 and 25-26).

Stemmed Wire Guides /ɪ/ (*i*t)

Lower tongue tip: shorter stem of double-ended wire guide used to position tongue tip behind Mandibular Central Incisors (31-41).

Raise tongue sides: tips of forked stemmed wire guide adjusted so tips touch alveolar ridge in approximate area of Maxillary Second Bicuspids and First Molars (15-16 and 25-26). The /ɪ/ (*i*t) appears to be slightly posterior to the /i/ (b*e*).

Groove tongue: shorter or longer stem of double-ended wire guide used to stroke mid-line of tip of tongue to encourage grooving.

Cue Sticks /ɪ/ (*i*t)

Cotton-tipped sticks dipped in cold water or parts of tongue depressors may be used to stimulate the same points for lingual contact as those given above.

/ɪ/ (*i*t) SELECTED PHONEME CHARACTERISTICS

DEVELOPMENTAL AGE:[1]

3 years

FREQUENCY OF OCCURRENCE OF PHONEME:[2]

9.22%; first in order of occurrence

VISUAL INTELLIGIBILITY:[3]
range—27% to 62%; composite 42%
VISUAL CONFUSION:[4]
/ɛ, ɪ, ʌ/ (b*e*t, *i*t, c*u*p)
AUDITORY INTELLIGIBILITY IN MILD-TO-SEVERE HEARING IMPAIRMENTS:[5]
80%
AUDITORY CONFUSION:[6]
/i, ɪ/ (b*e*, *i*t); /ɪ, ɛ, ʊ, ʌ, æ/ (*i*t, b*e*t, f*oo*t, c*u*p, *a*t)
RELATIVE PHONETIC POWER:[7]
260 (range of 1 to 680)
PHONEMIC CONFUSION:[8]
/ɪ/ (*i*t); /ə/ (sof*a*); /ɛ/ (b*e*t); /i/ (b*e*)
TYPICAL SPELLING:
a (cabb*a*ge); ae (*Ae*neas); *e* (pr*e*tty); *ee* (b*ee*n); *ei* (w*ei*rd); *ey* (all*ey*); *i* (*i*t); *ie* (s*ie*ve); *o* (w*o*men); *u* (b*u*sy); *ui* (b*ui*ld); *y* (h*y*mn)

/ɪ/ (*i*t) PRACTICE MATERIALS

The sound to be stimulated is /ɪ/ (*i*t). Only those words and phrases in which the respondent can articulate all of the sounds correctly, except for the target phoneme, should be utilized for practice. The same stimulation applies to the comparative practice materials provided at the end of this Section.

/h/ hit, hip, hear, hid; /p/ pick, pit, pin, pig; /b/ been, bit, big, bill; /t/ it, tip, Tim, 'til; /d/ Id, did, din, dip; /k/ kick, kin, kid, kit; /g/ give, gill, gear, given; /m/ mitt, mid, mill, miss; /n/ in, knit, nip, near; /hw/ whit, whim, which; /w/ wit, wig, wick, will; /f/ if, fit, fig, fin; /v/ vim, Vic, vicar; /θ/ thin, thing, think; /ð/ this, with, without; /s/ sit, sin, sip, Sid; /z/ is, zip, zipper; /ʃ/ ship, shin, shilling, shimmer; /tʃ/ itch, chin, chip, chick; /dʒ/ Jim, jip, jig, Jill; /l/ ill, lily, lit, limb; /r/ ear, rip, rig, rid; /j/ yip, year. *Phrases:* Give Bill the thin mitt. Did Tim tip this year? Jill hid the wig.

Stimulation Unit 3

Phonetic Symbol and Representative Word: /ɛ/ (b*e*t)

Symbol Systems
International Phonetic Alphabet: /ɛ/
Webster's New Collegiate Dictionary (1965): ĕ
Thorndike-Barnhardt Comprehensive Dictionary (1951): e, ã

[1-8] *Ibid.* (see p. 79).

Northampton Charts (Yale, 1946): -e-

Topographical Relationships of Phoneme Production

/ɛ/ (b*e*t) mid front lax unrounded

MANDIBLE:
slightly lower than for /ɪ/ (*i*t) and /e/ (v*a*cation)

LIPS:
more open than in preceding sounds

TONGUE:
Tip—at or near base of lower front teeth
Body—arched, with groove of arch slightly more depressed than for /ɪ/ (*i*t) and /e/ (v*a*cation)
Sides—remain in contact with maxillary molars.

AIR STREAM:
emitted through small opening between palate and tongue groove

NASAL PORT:
closed

VOCAL FOLDS:
vibrating

Stimulation Procedures

VISUAL-AUDITORY MODEL: A model demonstration is provided by the manipulation of the stimulator's face while the respondent observes. An auditory stimulus is usually given simultaneously as the stimulator is saying: "We are going to say /ɛ/ (b*e*t)." This step may be repeated.

STARTING POSITION. Respondent's articulators should be in the starting position before the manipulation is initiated: lips parted, mandible lowered slightly from position of closure, tongue in customary, relaxed position, vocal folds not vibrating.

SIMULTANEOUS STIMULATION. Stimulator places fingers in position on respondent's face. As the manipulation takes place, the respondent may observe the stimulator's face and/or hear an auditory stimulus.

EXTRAORAL MANIPULATION /ɛ/ (b*e*t)

1. Assume starting position.
2. Press tip of index finger on lower lip point 1.
3. Phonate.

If the above manipulation is not sufficient, use the additional manipulation procedures.

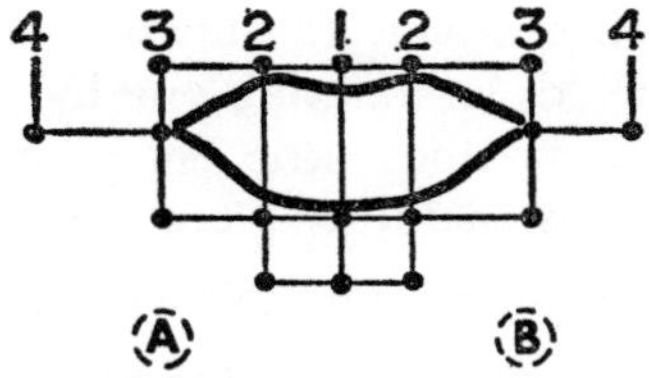

MANIPULATION MODEL: LIPS FORMAT.

ADDITIONAL MANIPULATION

1. Return to starting position.
2. While pressing index finger on lower lip point 1, oscillate fingertip for short intervals.
3. Simultaneously place thumb and middle finger of other hand on mid-lips points 3; gently and very slightly extend corners of lips.
4. Phonate. (The stimulator may signal phonation by placing little finger against respondent's larynx.)

/ɛ/ (b*e*t) Response Analysis and Extraoral Cues

MANDIBLE. If there is a tendency for the mandible to be lowered more than is appropriate for the /ɛ/ (b*e*t) sound, the little finger of the hand used to stimulate the lower lip may be hooked under the chin to prevent excessive mandibular depression. In some instances, the consonant following the vowel may have to be stimulated using the same mandibular position as for the vowel in order not to give a diphthongal quality to the vowel.

The mandible is slightly lower than for /e, ei) (v*a*cation, g*a*te). Description of /e/ (v*a*cation) and the manipulation for producing /e/ (v*a*cation) are given under the diphthong /ei/ (*a*ble) in Stimulation 12.

LIPS. Lips are still unrounded and are slightly more open than for /ɪ/ (*i*t) and /e/ (v*a*cation).

TONGUE. The groove in the arch of the tongue is more depressed and results in a wider opening above the tongue, both horizontally and laterally, in the /ɛ/ (b*e*t) sound than in the /ɪ/ (*i*t) and /e/ (v*a*cation).

NASAL PORT. If the airstream is being emitted through the nose, the stimulator may place the index finger under the nose of the respondent in order to indicate that the airstream is being improperly emitted.

The stimulator should accompany the tactile cue with the visual cue of shaking his head "no" or an *auditory* cue by saying "no."

VOCAL FOLDS. The stimulator's little finger may be placed against the respondent's larynx to signal phonation.

/ɛ/ (bet) PHONODENTAL GUIDES

Chapter 5 gives details concerning preparation and placement of phonodental guides. Figures 5 and 6 in Chapter 5 illustrate the approximate points of lingual contact for the guides.

Phonodental guides and intraoral cues may be used independently or in combination with the extraoral manipulations.

The extraoral manipulation is usually effective for eliciting this phoneme, and intraoral stimulation is not required. If intraoral stimulation is needed, one or more of the following phonodental guides may be utilized.

Denture Guides /ɛ/ (bet)

Denture guides are not usually utilized for identifying points of lingual contact, unless other sounds are involved. (See Figure 6.)

Dental Floss Guides /ɛ/ (bet)

Lower tongue tip: one knotted dental floss guide placed between Mandibular Central Incisors (31-41).

Raise tongue sides: two knotted dental floss guides placed between Maxillary Second Bicuspids and First Molars (15-16 and 25-26).

Stemmed Wire Guides /ɛ/ (bet)

Lower tongue tip: shorter stem of double-ended wire guide used to position tongue tip behind Mandibular Central Incisors (31-41).

Raise tongue sides: tips of forked stemmed wire guide adjusted so tips touch alveolar ridge in approximate area of Maxillary Second Bicuspids and First Molars (15-16 and 25-26). The /ɛ/ (bet) appears to be slightly posterior to the /ɪ/ (*i*t).

Cue Sticks /ɛ/ (bet)

Cotton-tipped sticks dipped in cold water or parts of tongue depressors may be used to stimulate the same points for lingual contact as those given above.

Note: This sound is moderately easy to stimulate.

/ɛ/ (bet) SELECTED PHONEME CHARACTERISTICS

DEVELOPMENTAL AGE:[1]

3 years

FREQUENCY OF OCCURRENCE OF PHONEME:[2]
2.92%; twelfth in order of occurrence
VISUAL INTELLIGIBILITY:[3]
range—27% to 50%; composite 38%
VISUAL CONFUSION:[4]
/ɛ, ɪ, ʌ/ (b*e*t, *i*t, c*u*p)
AUDITORY INTELLIGIBILITY IN MILD-TO-SEVERE HEARING IMPAIRMENTS:[5]
not given
AUDITORY CONFUSION:[6]
/ɪ, ɛ, ʊ, ʌ, æ/ (*i*t, b*e*t, f*oo*t, c*u*p, *a*t)
/ei, æ, ɛ, ɑ/ (g*a*te, *a*t, b*e*t, l*o*t and c*a*lm)
RELATIVE PHONETIC POWER:[7]
350 (range of 1 to 680)
PHONEMIC CONFUSION:[8]
/ɛ/ (b*e*t); /ɪ/ (*i*t); /a/ (l*a*—French article);
/æ/ (*a*t); /e/ (v*a*cation)
TYPICAL SPELLING:
a (*a*ny); *a* (re) (r*a*re); *ae* (*ae*rial); *ai* (s*ai*d); *ai* (*r*) (*ai*r); *ay* (s*ay*s); *e* (*e*lbow); *ea* (br*ea*d); *ei* (h*ei*fer); *ei* (*r*) (th*ei*r); *eo* (l*eo*pard); *ie* (fr*ie*nd); *oe* (asaf*oe*tida); *u* (b*u*ry); *ue* (g*ue*ss)

/ɛ/ (b*e*t) PRACTICE MATERIALS

The sound to be stimulated is /ɛ/ (b*e*t). Only those words and phrases in which the respondent can articulate all of the sounds correctly, except for the target phoneme, should be utilized for practice. The same stipulation applies to the practice materials provided at the end of this Section.

/h/ hen, hem, head, heifer; /p/ pep, pet, peg, pen; /b/ ebb, bed, Ben, bet, beg; /t/ Etta, Ted, ten; /d/ Ed, debt, deaf, dead; /k/ echo, keg, kettle, Ked; /g/ egg, get, guess, again; /m/ "m," Emma, met, men; /n/ "n," net, Ned, never; /hw/ when, whet, whether, where; /w/ wet, wed, web, well; /f/ "f," Effie, fed, fell; /v/ every, ever, event, vent; /θ/ Ethel, ethics; /ð/ their, them, then; /s/ "s," sent, said, says, senate; /z/ zep, Zen, Zell; /ʃ/ shell, shed, shelf, shepherd; /tʃ/ etch, wretch, check, Cheddar; /dʒ/ edge, gem, jet, Jess; /l/ "l," let, Ellen, left; /r/ err, red, wreck, wren; /j/ yen, yell, yet, yes. *Phrases:* Emma has a yellow bell. Ed met ten men. Send them ten gems.

[1-8] *Ibid.* (see p. 79).

Stimulation Unit 4

Phonetic Symbol and Representative Word: /æ/ (*a*t)

Symbol Systems

International Phonetic Alphabet: /æ/
Webster's New Collegiate Dictionary (1965): ă
Thorndike-Barnhardt Comprehensive Dictionary (1951): a
Northampton Charts (Yale, 1946): -a-

Topographical Relationships of Phoneme Production
/æ/ (*a*t) low front tense unrounded

MANDIBLE:
slightly more depressed than for /ɛ/
LIPS:
continue to follow passively the depression of mandible
TONGUE:
Tip—at or near base of lower front teeth
Body—continues downward and backward movement
Sides—complete separation from maxillary teeth
AIRSTREAM:
passes over the tongue that lies almost flat on floor of mouth cavity
NASAL PORT:
closed
VOCAL FOLDS:
vibrating

Stimulation Procedures

VISUAL-AUDITORY MODEL. A model demonstration is provided by the manipulation of the stimulator's face while the respondent observes. An auditory stimulus is usually given simultaneously as the stimulator is saying: "We are going to say /æ/ (*a*t)." This step may be repeated.

STARTING POSITION. Respondent's articulators should be in the starting position before the manipulation is initiated: lips parted; mandible lowered slightly from position of closure; tongue in customary, relaxed position; vocal folds not vibrating.

SIMULTANEOUS STIMULATION. Stimulator places fingers in position on respondent's face. As the manipulation takes place, the respondent may observe the stimulator's face and/or hear an auditory stimulus.

EXTRAORAL MANIPULATION /æ/ (*a*t)

1. Assume starting position.

2. Place thumb and middle finger on lower lip points 2.
3. Lower mandible slightly more than for /ɛ/ (b*e*t).
4. Press lip points 2 with thumb and middle finger and move halfway to mid-lip points 3.
5. Phonate.

If the above manipulation is not sufficient, use the additional manipulation procedures.

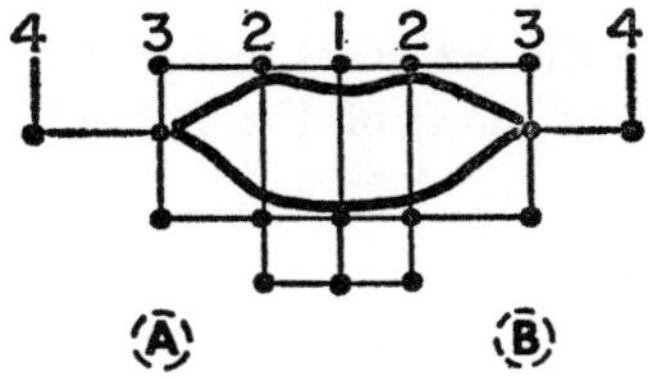

MANIPULATION MODEL: LIPS FORMAT.

ADDITIONAL MANIPULATION

1. Return to starting position.
2. Repeatedly slide thumb and middle finger simultaneously between lower lip point 2 toward mid-lip point 3.
3. Phonate. (The stimulators may signal phonation by placing little finger against respondent's larynx.)

/æ/ (*a*t) Response Analysis and Extraoral Cues

MANDIBLE. If there is a tendency for the mandible to be lowered more than is appropriate for the /æ/ (*a*t) sound, the little finger of the hand used to stimulate the lower lip may be hooked under the chin to prevent excessive mandibular depression. If mandible and body of tongue are too high, there is a distortion of resonance in the form of nasality. If such distortion occurs, both tongue and mandible should be lowered.

LIPS. The lips are not rounded. The mouth opening is wider than for any other front vowels studied.

TONGUE. The tongue should break bilateral contact with the upper molars. There is a greater difference between the positions of the tongue for /ɛ/ (b*e*t) and /æ/ (*a*t) than for any other two adjacent front sounds in English. The respondent should avoid humping the tongue.

NASAL PORT. If the airstream is being emitted through the nose, the stimulator can place the index finger under the nose of the respondent in order to indicate that the airstream is being improperly emitted. The stimulator should accompany the *tactile* cue with the *visual* cue of shaking his head "no" or an *auditory* cue by saying "no."

VOCAL FOLDS. The stimulator's little finger may be placed against the respondent's larynx to signal phonation.

/æ/ (*a*t) PHONODENTAL GUIDES

Chapter 5 gives details concerning preparation and placement of phonodental guides. Figures 5 and 6 in Chapter 5 illustrate the points of lingual contact for the guides.

Phonodental guides and intraoral cues may be used independently or in combination with the extraoral manipulations. If intraoral stimulation is needed, one or more of the following phonodental guides may be utilized.

Denture Guides /æ/ (*a*t)

Denture guides are not usually utilized for identifying points of lingual contact for /æ/ (*a*t).

Dental Floss Guides /æ/ (*a*t)

Lower tongue tip: one knotted dental floss guide placed between Mandibular Central Incisors (31-41); or two knotted dental floss guides between Mandibular Cuspids and First Bicuspids (33-34 and 43-44).

Stemmed Wire Guides /æ/ (*a*t)

Lower tongue tip: shorter stem of double-ended wire guide used to position tongue tip behind Mandibular Incisors (31-41).

Lower tongue body: stemmed reflexor used to stimulate body of tongue so it will assume low position by touching tongue tip lightly or by gently drawing reflexor along midline.

Cue Sticks /æ/ (*a*t)

Cotton-tipped sticks dipped in cold water or parts of tongue depressors may be used to stimulate the same points for lingual contact as those given above.

/æ/ (*a*t) SELECTED PHONEME CHARACTERISTICS

DEVELOPMENTAL AGE:[1]
3 years

FREQUENCY OF OCCURRENCE OF PHONEME:[2]
2.00%; nineteenth in order of occurrence

VISUAL INTELLIGIBILITY:[3]
range—16% to 27%; composite 44%

VISUAL CONFUSION:[4]
not given

AUDITORY INTELLIGIBILITY IN MILD-TO-SEVERE HEARING IMPAIRMENTS:[5]
75%

AUDITORY CONFUSION:[6]

/ɔi, ɔ, ɑi, æ/ (b*oy*, s*aw*, m*i*ce, *a*t)

/ɪ, ɛ, ʊ, ʌ, æ/ (*i*t, b*e*t, f*oo*t, c*u*p, *a*t)

/ei, æ, ɛ, ɑ/ (g*a*te, *a*t, b*e*t, l*o*t and c*a*lm)

RELATIVE PHONETIC POWER:[7]

490 (range of 1 to 680)

PHONEMIC CONFUSION:[8]

/æ/ (*a*t); /ɛ/ (b*e*t); /e/ (v*a*cation); /a/ (l*a*—French article)

TYPICAL SPELLING:

a (*a*t); *ai* (pl*ai*d); *al* (s*al*mon); *au* (*au*nt); *i* (mer*i*ngue)

/æ/ (*a*t) PRACTICE MATERIALS

The sound to be stimulated is /æ/ (*a*t). Only those words and phrases in which the respondent can articulate all of the sounds correctly, except for the target phoneme, should be utilized for practice. The same stipulation applies to the practice materials provided at the end of this Section.

/h/ hat, has, had, Hal; /p/ pack, pat, path, pan; /b/ ban, bat, bass, bath; /d/ add, dad, Dan, dash; /k/ cap, cat, can, cash; /g/ Aggie, gag, gal, gas, /m/ am, mat, man, mad; /n/ an, Nan, gnat, Nash; /f/ fad, fan, fat, fashion; /v/ Van, vat, Val; /θ/ thank, bath, math, lath; /ð/ that, fathom, than; /s/ sat, sad, Sam; /z/ as, has, dazzle, Zach; /ʃ/ ash, shack, passion, dash; /ʒ/ azure, jabot, casual; /tʃ/ chap, chat, attach, match; /dʒ/ adage, Japan, jazz, badge; /l/ Al, pal, Sally, lad; /r/ ram, ran, rat, rap; /j/ yak, yam, yank, yap. *Phrases:* Pat had a hat. Sam's badge. Thank Aggie. Nan's cat can catch a rat.

COMPARATIVE PRACTICE MATERIALS

SECTION A: FRONT VOWELS

The sounds to be stimulated are /i, ɪ, ɛ, æ/ (b*e*, *i*t, b*e*t, *a*t). Only those words and phrases in which the respondent can articulate all of the sounds correctly, except for the target phoneme, should be utilized for practice.

	/i/ (b*e*)	/ɪ/ (*i*t)	/ɛ/ (b*e*t)	/æ/ (*a*t)
INITIAL POSITION:	eat	it	Etta	at
	eerie	ear	elf	am

[1-8] *Ibid.* (see p. 79).

MEDIAL POSITION:	deed	did	dead	dad
	feed		fed	fad
	ream	rit	red	rat
	neat	knit	net	gnat
	meet	mitt	met	mat
	seat	sit	set	sat
	cheap	chip	chair	chat
	keen	kin	ken	can
FINAL POSITION:	me	Amy	heh	baa
	Lee	Sally		

SECTION B: BACK VOWELS

Representative Words:	b*oo*t	f*oo*t	s*aw*, w*a*r	c*a*lm, l*o*t
International Phonetic Alphabet:	/u/	/ʊ/	/ɔ/	/ɑ/
Webster's New Collegiate Dictionary (1965):	ü	u̇	ȯ	ä
Thorndike-Barnhardt Comprehensive Dictionary (1951):	ü	u̇	ô	ä, o
Northampton Charts (Yale, 1946):	oo (1)	oo (2)	aw	a(r)

Stimulation Units are provided for the four back vowels. These include the high back, tense, rounded /u/ (b*oo*t), high back, lax, rounded /ʊ/ (f*oo*t), mid back, lax, rounded /ɔ/ (s*aw*), and low back, lax, unrounded /ɑ/ (c*a*lm, l*o*t). The mid back, tense, rounded /o/ (*o*bey) is discussed under the diphthong /ou/ (g*o*) in Stimulation Unit 13.

The four back vowels that are to be discussed, like the front vowels, have certain characteristics in common. The tongue, lips, and mandible play important roles. The movement of the mandible is practically the same as for the front vowels in that the depression for the opposite front and back vowels is practically the same; the lips reverse the order of opening in that they are rounded and protruded for the high back tense /u/ (b*oo*t) sound and unpursed appreciably as the mandible drops to its lowest back position for /ɑ/ (c*a*lm, l*o*t). The tongue body moves to a posterior, superior position and is pulled distally from the position it assumed for the front vowels. The apex of the tongue is no longer important.

With the low back /ɑ/ (c*a*lm, l*o*t) sound, there is no contact of the lateral borders of the tongue with maxillary teeth. In the continued elevation of the mandible, the tongue arch produces /o/ (*o*bey). With continued elevation, the sound /ʊ/ (f*oo*t) is produced. For the highest back sound /u/ (b*oo*t), the mandible is elevated to a rest position, and the lateral borders of the tongue are in contact with the maxillary teeth for /o, ʊ, u/ (*o*bey, f*oo*t, b*oo*t). With the low back /ɔ/ (*saw, war*) and /ɑ/ (c*a*lm, l*o*t) sounds, there is no contact of the lateral borders of the tongue with the maxillary teeth.

All examples of pronunciations used in this book are standard pronunciations. Individual pronunciations may vary from area to area. If acceptable pronunciations differ, a substitute word may be used in a given exercise.

Stimulation Unit 5

Phonetic Symbol and Representative Word: /u/ (b*oo*t)

Symbol Systems

International Phonetic Alphabet: /u/
Webster's New Collegiate Dictionary (1965): ü
Thorndike-Barnhardt Comprehensive Dictionary (1951): ü
Northampton Charts (Yale, 1946): $\overset{1}{\text{oo}}$

Topographical Relationships of Phoneme Production
/u/ (b*oo*t) high back tense rounded

MANDIBLE:
at highest position for the back vowels
LIPS:
closely rounded and protruded
TONGUE:
Tip—depressed and retracted
Body—high and back
Sides—in contact with maxillary molars
AIRSTREAM:
emitted through small opening between palate and tongue
NASAL PORT:
closed
VOCAL FOLDS:
vibrating

Stimulation Procedures

VISUAL-AUDITORY MODEL. A model demonstration is provided by the manipulation of the stimulator's face while the respondent observes. An auditory stimulus is usually given simultaneously as the stimulator is saying: "We are going to say /u/ (b*oo*t)." This step may be repeated.

STARTING POSITION. Respondent's articulators should be in the starting position before the manipulation is initiated: lips parted, mandible lowered slightly from position of closure, tongue in customary relaxed position, vocal folds not vibrating.

SIMULTANEOUS STIMULATION. Stimulator places fingers in position on respondent's face. As the manipulation takes place, the respondent may observe the stimulator's face and/or hear an auditory stimulus.

EXTRAORAL MANIPULATION /u/ (b*oo*t)

1. Assume starting position.
2. Place thumb and middle finger on mid-lip points 3.
3. Direct the corners of the mouth toward mid-lip line 1, forming a small rounded opening.
4. Phonate after lips have assumed rounded position.

If the above manipulation is not sufficient, use the additional manipulation procedures.

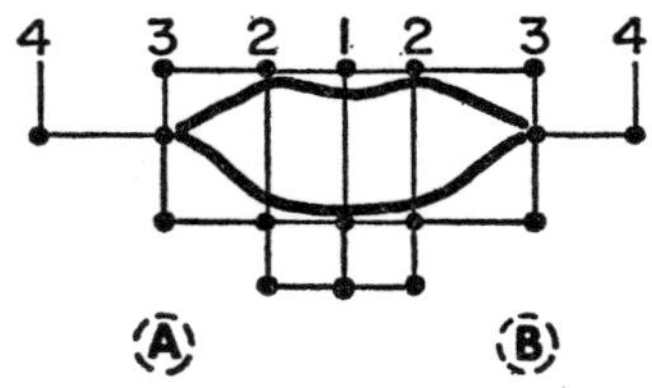

MANIPULATION MODEL: LIPS FORMAT.

ADDITIONAL MANIPULATION

1. Return to starting position.
2. Place thumb and middle finger of *both hands* adjacent to mid-lip points 3.
3. Direct the corners and sides of the mouth toward mid-lip line 1—forming a small rounded opening.
4. Phonate after lips have assumed rounded position. (The stimulator may signal phonation by placing little finger against respondent's larynx.)

/u/ (b*oo*t) Response Analysis and Extraoral Cues

MANDIBLE. The mandible is lowered to approximately the same degree as for /i/ (b*e*).

LIPS. The /u/ (b*oo*t) is the most tense and rounded of the back vowels. During production, the lips continue to round. Too large an opening may produce an /o/ (*o*bey). If tongue tip is elevated, a sound approaching an unrounded /i/ (b*e*) will be produced. Care should be taken that the lips do not protrude too much after the production of the sound is mastered. Lips should not be too tense, and the upper lip should not be drawn downward.

TONGUE. During the production of the /u/ (b*oo*t), the back of the tongue is at its highest position. Because of the high back position, some respondents tend to add a /k/ (*k*eep) or a /g/ (*g*o) sound. If this type of error occurs, the /u/ (b*oo*t) should be taught in isolation until production is firmly established. A pause should be used between the /u/ (b*oo*t) and the following sounds until no interference by extraneous sounds occurs.

AIRSTREAM. Too much breath emitted on the /u/ (b*oo*t) impairs the resonance.

NASAL PORT. If the airstream is being emitted through the nose, the stimulator can place the index finger under the nose of the respondent in order to indicate that the airstream is being improperly emitted. The stimulator should accompany the *tactile* cue with the *visual* cue of shaking his head "no" or an *auditory* cue by saying "no."

VOCAL FOLDS. The stimulator's little finger may be placed against the respondent's larynx to signal phonation.

/u/ (b*oo*t) PHONODENTAL GUIDES

Chapter Five gives details concerning preparation and placement of phonodental guides. Figures 5 and 6 in Chapter 5 illustrate the approximate points of lingual contact for the guides.

Phonodental guides and intraoral cues may be used independently or in combination with the extraoral manipulations.

The extraoral manipulation is usually effective for eliciting this phoneme, and intraoral stimulation is not required. If intraoral stimulation is needed, one or more of the following phonodental guides may be utilized.

Denture Guides /u/ (boot)

Denture guides are not usually utilized for identifying points of lingual contact, unless other sounds are involved. If so, use position in approximate area of Maxillary First Molars and Second Molars (16-17 and 26-27). (See Figure 6.)

Raise tongue sides: two knotted dental floss guides placed between Maxillary First Molars and Second Molars (16-17 and 26-27). The deeper within the oral cavity the knotted dental floss guides must be located, the more difficult they are to place. The use of the forked stemmed guide is recommended.

Stemmed Wire Guides /u/ (b*oo*t)

Raise tongue sides: tips of forked stemmed wire guide adjusted so tips touch alveolar ridge in approximate area of Maxillary First Molars and Second Molars (16-17 and 26-27).

Cue Sticks /u/ (b*oo*t)

Cotton-tipped sticks dipped in cold water or parts of tongue depressors may be used to stimulate the same points for lingual contact as those given above.

Note: This sound is easily stimulated and is one of the basic vowels used in syllables and words for stimulating target consonant sounds.

/u/ (b*oo*t) SELECTED PHONEME CHARACTERISTICS

DEVELOPMENTAL AGE:[1]

3 years

FREQUENCY OF OCCURRENCE OF PHONEME:[2]

1.20%; thirty-third in order of occurrence

VISUAL INTELLIGIBILITY:[3]

range—53% to 100%; composite 66%

VISUAL CONFUSION:[4]

not given

AUDITORY INTELLIGIBILITY IN MILD-TO-SEVERE HEARING IMPAIRMENTS:[5]

95%

AUDITORY CONFUSION:[6]

/u, ou/ (b*oo*t, g*o*); /ou, u, ɔ/ (g*o*, b*oo*t, s*aw* and w*ar*)

RELATIVE PHONETIC POWER:[7]

310 (range 1 to 680)

PHONEMIC CONFUSION:[8]

/u/ (b*oo*t); /hw/ (*wh*at); /w/ (*w*e); /ʊ/ (f*oo*t); /o/ (*o*bey)

TYPICAL SPELLING:

eu (rh*eu*matic); *eu* (kn*ew*); *ieu* (l*ieu*); *ioux* (S*ioux*); *o* (m*o*ve); *oe* (can*oe*); *oo* (t*oo*); *ou* (cr*ou*p); *ough* (thr*ough*); *ous* (rendezv*ous*); *u* (r*u*le); *ue* (d*ue*); *uh* (b*uh*l); *ui* (fr*ui*t); *wo* (t*wo*)

/u/ (b*oo*t) PRACTICE MATERIALS

The sound to be stimulated is /u/ (b*oo*t). Only those words and phrases in which the respondent can articulate all of the sounds correctly, except for the target phoneme, should be utilized for practice.

[1-8] *Ibid.* (see p. 79).

The same stipulation applies to the practice materials provided at the end of this Section. /h/ who, hoop, hoot, hoof; /p/ pooh, poor, pool, prove; /b/ boo, bamboo, boom, boot; /t/ too, tattoo, tool, into; /d/ do, undo, doom, dude; /k/ coo, crew, coon, cool; /g/ goo, grew, goose; /m/ moo, moon, move, moose; /n/ new, canoe, noon, noose; /hw/ whoop, whoopee; /w/ woo, wooed, wooes; /f/ flew, Fu Manchu, food, fool; /v/ voodoo; /θ/ Matthew, tooth, booth; /s/ Sue, Sioux, soon, soup; /z/ ooze, zoo, zoom, Zulu; /ʃ/ shoe, shoo, shoot, sure; /ʒ/ Bijou; /tʃ/ chew, chewed, choose; /dʒ/ Jew, June, jewel, juice; /l/ oolong, igloo, lieu, Lucy; /r/ rue, room, root, rude; /j/ you, youth, your, you'd. *Phrases:* Whose booth? Poor Lucy. Schoolroom rule.

Stimulation Unit 6

Phonetic Symbol and Representative Word: /ʊ/ (f*oo*t)

Symbol Systems

International Phonetic Alphabet: /ʊ/
Webster's New Collegiate Dictionary (1965): u̇
Thorndike-Barnhardt Comprehensive Dictionary (1951): u̇
Northampton Charts (Yale, 1946): $\overset{2}{\text{oo}}$

Topographical Relationships of Phoneme Production
/ʊ/ (f*oo*t) high back lax rounded

MANDIBLE:
high, almost closed, allowing only a slight opening between upper and lower teeth

LIPS:
rounded with less protrusion than for /u/ (b*oo*t)

TONGUE:
Tip—retracted
Body—arched upwards and backwards toward velum
Sides—in contact with maxillary molars

AIRSTREAM:
emitted through small opening between palate and tongue

NASAL PORT:
closed

VOCAL FOLDS:
vibrating

Stimulation Procedures

VISUAL-AUDITORY MODEL. A model demonstration is provided by the manipulation of the stimulator's face while the respondent observes. An auditory stimulus is usually given simultaneously as the stimulator is saying: "We are going to say /ʊ/ (f*oo*t)." This step may be repeated.

STARTING POSITION. Respondent's articulators should be in the starting position before the manipulation is initiated: lips parted, mandible lowered slightly from position of closure, tongue in customary, relaxed position, vocal folds not vibrating.

SIMULTANEOUS STIMULATION. Stimulator places fingers in position on respondent's face. As the manipulation takes place, the respondent may observe the stimulator's face and/or hear an auditory stimulus.

EXTRAORAL MANIPULATION /ʊ/ (f*oo*t)

1. Assume starting position.
2. Place thumb and middle finger of one hand just above mid-lip points 3.
3. Place thumb and middle finger of other hand just below mid-lip points 3.
4. Bring lips into rounded position with protrusion.
5. Phonate.

If the above manipulation is not sufficient, use the additional manipulation procedures.

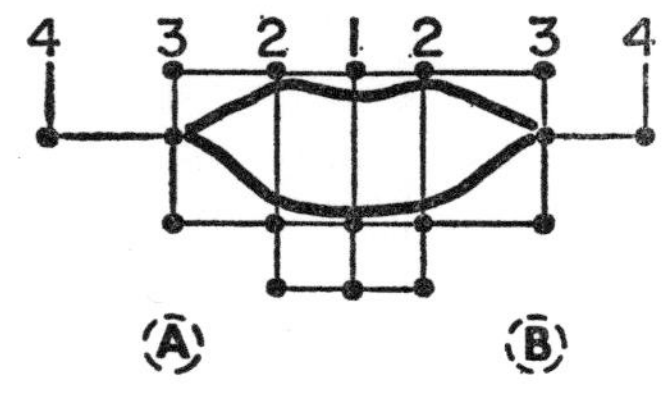

MANIPULATION MODEL: LIPS FORMAT.

ADDITIONAL MANIPULATION

1. Return to starting position.
2. With the thumb and middle finger of one hand, push the lips toward the midline in order to obtain the rounded protrusion.
3. With the thumb and middle finger of the other hand, extend the corners of the mouth at midline points 3 so that too much rounding will not occur and produce /u/ (b*oo*t).
4. It is sometimes helpful to push against the lower mandible as lips assume a vertical, elongated oval shape.
5. Phonate. (The stimulator may signal phonation by placing little finger against respondent's larynx.)

/ʊ/ (f*oo*t) Response Analysis and Extraoral Cues

MANDIBLE. If there is a tendency for the mandible to be lowered more than is appropriate for the /ʊ/ (f*oo*t) sound, the little finger of the hand used to stimulate the lower lip may be hooked under the chin to prevent excessive mandibular depression.

LIPS. Lip rounding is an important difference between /ʊ/ (f*oo*t) and /u/ (b*oo*t). The former has less rounding than the latter. Unrounding the lips will produce a centralized or fronted sound approximating /ʌ/ (c*u*p) or /ɪ/ (*i*t).

TONGUE. The tongue position for the /ʊ/ (f*oo*t) is considered lower than for /u/ (b*oo*t), but a change from one sound to the other can be made with little tongue movement.

NASAL PORT. If the airstream is being emitted through the nose, the stimulator can place the index finger under the nose of the respondent in order to indicate that the airstream is being improperly emitted. The stimulator should accompany the *tactile* cue with the *visual* cue of shaking his head "no" or an *auditory* cue by saying "no."

VOCAL FOLDS. The stimulator's little finger may be placed against the respondent's larynx to signal phonation.

/ʊ/ (f*oo*t) PHONODENTAL GUIDES

Chapter Five gives details concerning preparation and placement of phonodental guides. Figures 5 and 6 in Chapter 5 illustrate the approximate points of lingual contact for the guides.

Phonodental guides and intraoral cues may be used independently or in combination with the extraoral manipulations. If intraoral stimulation is needed, one or more of the following phonodental guides may be utilized.

Denture Guides /ʊ/ (f*oo*t)

Denture guides are not usually utilized for identifying points of lingual contact, unless other sounds are involved. If so, use position in approximate area of Maxillary First Molars and Second Molars (16-17 and 26-27). (See Figure 6.)

Dental Floss Guides /ʊ/ (f*oo*t)

Raise tongue sides: two knotted dental floss guides placed between Maxillary First Molars and Second Molars (16-17 and 26-27). The deeper within the oral cavity the knotted dental floss guides must be located, the more difficult they are to place. The use of the forked stemmed guide is recommended.

Stemmed Wire Guides /ʊ/ (f*oo*t)

Raise tongue sides: tips of forked stemmed wire guide adjusted so tips touch alveolar ridge in approximate area of Maxillary First Molars and Second Molars (16-17 and 26-27).

Cue Sticks /ʊ/ (f*oo*t)

Cotton-tipped sticks dipped in cold water or parts of tongue depressors may be used to stimulate the same points for lingual contact as those given above.

/ʊ/ (f*oo*t) SELECTED PHONEME CHARACTERISTICS

DEVELOPMENTAL AGE:[1]
3 years

FREQUENCY OF OCCURRENCE OF PHONEME:[2]
1.53%; twenty-fifth in order of occurrence

VISUAL INTELLIGIBILITY:[3]
range—20% to 50%; composite 46%

VISUAL CONFUSION:[4]
/ɔ/ (s*aw*), /ʊ/ (f*oo*t)

AUDITORY INTELLIGIBILITY IN MILD-TO-SEVERE HEARING IMPAIRMENTS:[5]
92%

AUDITORY CONFUSION:[6]
/ɪ, ɛ, ʊ, ʌ, æ/ (*i*t, b*e*t, f*oo*t, c*u*p, *a*t)

RELATIVE PHONETIC POWER:[7]
460 (range of 1 to 680)

PHONEMIC CONFUSION:[8]
/ʊ/ (f*oo*t), /u/ (b*oo*t) /w/ (*w*e), /ɝ/ (b*ir*d)

TYPICAL SPELLING:
o (w*o*lf); *oo* (h*oo*k); *ou* (w*ou*ld); *u* (f*u*ll); *or* (w*or*sted)

/ʊ/ (f*oo*t) PRACTICE MATERIALS

The sound to be stimulated is /ʊ/ (f*oo*t). Only those words and phrases in which the respondent can articulate all of the sounds correctly, except for the target phoneme, should be utilized for practice. The same stipulation applies to the practice materials provided at the end of this Section.

/h/ hood, hook, hoof; /p/ put, pudding; /b/ book, bushel; /t/ took, put; /d/ could; /k/ cook, crook, shook; /g/ good; /w/ wood; /f/ full, foot; /s/ stood, soot, puss; /ʊ/ should, shook, bush; /l/ look, full; /r/ rook. *Phrases:* Look at the book. He took the cookies. She looked for good wool.

[1-8] *Ibid.* (see p. 79).

Stimulation Unit 7

Phonetic Symbol and Representative Words: /ɔ/ (*saw*, w*a*r)

Symbol Systems

International Phonetic Alphabet: /ɔ/
Webster's New Collegiate Dictionary (1965): ȯ
Thorndike-Barnhardt Comprehensive Dictionary (1951): ô
Northampton Charts (Yale, 1946): aw

Topographical Relationships of Phoneme Production
/ɔ/ (*saw*, w*a*r) mid back lax rounded

MANDIBLE:
only slightly lower than for /ʊ/ (f*oo*t) and /o/ (*o*bey)
LIPS:
open, slightly rounded, little protrusion
TONGUE:
Tip—near base of lower front teeth
Body—arched upward and backward toward velum
Sides—complete separation from maxillary teeth
AIRSTREAM:
emitted through opening between tongue and palate
NASAL PORT:
closed
VOCAL FOLDS:
vibrating

Stimulation Procedures

VISUAL-AUDITORY MODEL. A model demonstration is provided by the manipulation of the stimulator's face while the respondent observes. An auditory stimulus is usually given simultaneously as the stimulator is saying: "We are going to say /ɔ/ (*saw*, w*a*r)." This step may be repeated.

STARTING POSITION. Respondent's articulators should be in the starting position before the manipulation is initiated: lips parted, mandible lowered slightly from position of closure, tongue in customary, relaxed position, vocal folds not vibrating.

SIMULTANEOUS STIMULATION. Stimulator places fingers in position on respondent's face. As the manipulation takes place, the respondent may observe the stimulator's face and/or hear an auditory stimulus.

EXTRAORAL MANIPULATION /ɔ/ (s*aw*, w*a*r)

1. Assume starting position.
2. Place thumb and middle finger of one hand on mid-lip points 3.
3. Shape lips into slightly oval form.
4. Place thumb and middle finger of other hand on lower lip points 2.
5. Lower mandible slightly.
6. Shape lips into slightly oval form with the lower hand.
7. Phonate.

If the above manipulation is not sufficient, use the additional manipulation procedures.

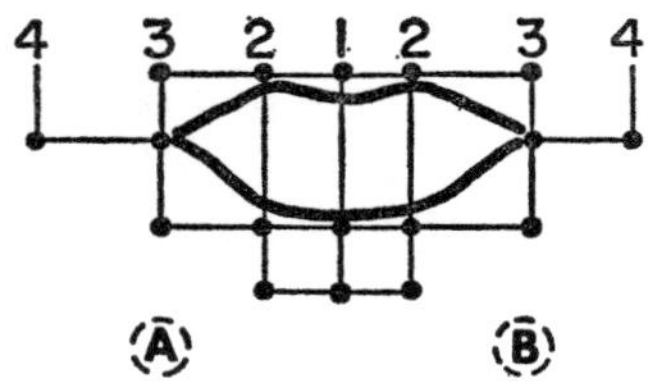

MANIPULATION MODEL: LIPS FORMAT.

ADDITIONAL MANIPULATION

1. Return to the starting position.
2. If the oval shape is not achieved with the above manipulation, the sides of thumb and the other fingers of one hand may be utilized to push the corners of the lips toward the mid-lip line.
3. Phonate. (The stimulator may signal phonation by placing little finger against respondent's larynx.)

Note: The procedures may be reversed so that the /ɑ/ (c*a*lm, l*o*t) is stimulated and the shaping of the lips for /ɔ/ (s*aw*, w*a*r) takes place while the /ɑ/ (c*a*lm, l*o*t) is being produced.

/ɔ/ (s*aw*, w*a*r) Response Analysis and Extraoral Cues

MANDIBLE. The /ɔ/ (s*aw*, w*a*r) sound is produced with the mandible slightly lower than for the /ʊ/ (f*oo*t) sound. If mandible is lowered too much, support it with the little finger.

LIPS. The /ɔ/ (s*aw*, w*a*r) has less lip tension than the /ʊ/ (f*oo*t). The most significant difference between them is the greater amount of lip rounding on /ʊ/ (f*oo*t) and greater depression of the mandible for the /ɔ/ (s*aw*, w*a*r).

TONGUE. The /ɔ/ (s*aw*, w*a*r) sound uses less tongue tension than the /ʊ/ (f*oo*t). The tongue position is slightly more relaxed. The tongue is no longer in contact with the mandibular teeth.

NASAL PORT. If the airstream is being emitted through the nose, the stimulator can place the index finger under the nose of the respondent in order to indicate that the airstream is being improperly emitted. The stimulator should accompany the *tactile* cue with the *visual* cue of shaking his head "no" or an *auditory* cue by saying "no."

VOCAL FOLDS. The stimulator's little finger may be placed against the respondent's larynx to signal phonation.

/ɔ/ (*saw*, w*a*r) PHONODENTAL GUIDES

Chapter 5 gives details concerning preparation and placement of phonodental guides. Figures 5 and 6 in Chapter 5 illustrate the approximate points of lingual contact for the guides.

Phonodental guides and intraoral cues may be used independently or in combination with the extraoral manipulations. If intraoral stimulation is needed, one or more of the following phonodental guides may be utilized.

Stemmed Wire Guides /ɔ/ (*saw*, w*a*r)

Lower tongue body: stemmed reflexor used to stimulate body of tongue so it will assume low position by touching tongue tip lightly or by gently drawing reflexor along midline.

Cue Sticks /ɔ/ (*saw*, w*a*r)

Cotton-tipped sticks dipped in cold water or parts of tongue depressors may be used to stimulate the same points for lingual contact as those given above.

/ɔ/ (*saw*, w*a*r) SELECTED PHONEME CHARACTERISTICS

DEVELOPMENTAL AGE:[1]

3 years

FREQUENCY OF OCCURRENCE OF PHONEME:[2]

2.13%; sixteenth in order of occurrence

VISUAL INTELLIGIBILITY:[3]

range—50% to 100%; composite 68%

VISUAL CONFUSION:[4]

/ɔ/ (*saw*), /ʊ/ (f*oo*t)

AUDITORY INTELLIGIBILITY IN MILD-TO-SEVERE HEARING IMPAIRMENTS:[5]

83%

AUDITORY CONFUSION:[6]

/ɔi, ɔ, ɑi, æ/ (b*oy*, *saw* and w*a*r, m*i*ce, *a*t); /ei, ɑi, ɔ/ (g*a*te, m*i*ce, *saw* and w*a*r)

RELATIVE PHONETIC POWER:[7]

680 (range of 1 to 680)

PHONEMIC CONFUSION:[8]
/ɔ/ (*saw*, w*a*r); /o/ (*o*bey); /ɑ/ (c*a*lm, l*o*t)
TYPICAL SPELLING:
a (*a*ll); *ah* (Ut*ah*); *al* (w*al*k); *as* (Arkans*as*); *au* (*au*tomobile); *aw* (*aw*l); *awe* (*awe*); *o* (*o*rder); *oa* (br*oa*d); *oi* (reserv*oi*r); *ou* (*ou*ght)

/ɔ/ (*saw*, w*a*r) PRACTICE MATERIALS

The sound to be stimulated is /ɔ/ (*saw*, w*a*r). Only those words and phrases in which the respondent can articulate all of the sounds correctly, except for the target phoneme, should be utilized for practice. The same stipulation applies to the practice materials provided at the end of this Section.

/h/ haw, hawl, hawk; /p/ paw, Paul; /b/ ball, bought, daub; /t/ tall, aught, tawny; /d/ awed, daub, pawed, dawn; /k/ auk, caw, cough, caught; /g/ auger, augment, gawk, guffaw; /m/ maul, maw, Maude; /n/ awning, gnaw, naughty, naught; /ŋ/ wrong, strong; /hw/ wharf; /w/ wall, Waugh, warm, awkward; /f/ awful, fall, fawn, fought; /v/ Vaughn, vault; /θ/ authority, thaw, author, thaws; /ð/ moths; /s/ Australia, saw, sauce, sawed; /z/ laws, gauze; /ʃ/ Shaw, shawl; /tʃ/ chalk; /dʒ/ jaw, jaundice; /l/ awl, law, call, ball; /r/ aura, raw, Raleigh, lord; /j/ jaw. *Phrases:* Maude saw the chalk. Paul bought a saw and an auger. Shaw bought the ball.

Stimulation Unit 8

Phonetic Symbol and Representative Word: /ɑ/ (c*a*lm, l*o*t)

Symbol Systems

International Phonetic Alphabet: /ɑ/
Webster's New Collegiate Dictionary (1965): ä
Thorndike-Barnhardt Comprehensive Dictionary (1951): ä, o
Northampton Charts (Yale, 1946: a(r), -o-

Topographical Relationships of Phoneme Production
/ɑ/ (c*a*lm, l*o*t) low back lax unrounded

MANDIBLE:
dropped to lowest back position
LIPS:
passive and unrounded, presenting largest opening for any vowel

[1-8] *Ibid.* (see p. 79).

TONGUE:
neutral position, practically flat on floor of mouth
AIRSTREAM:
emitted through mouth
NASAL PORT:
closed
VOCAL FOLDS:
vibrating

Stimulation Procedures

VISUAL-AUDITORY MODEL. A model demonstration is provided by the manipulation of the stimulator's face while the respondent observes. An auditory stimulus is usually given simultaneously as the stimulator is saying: "We are going to say /ɑ/ (c**a**lm, l**o**t)." This step may be repeated.

STARTING POSITION. Respondent's articulators should be in the starting position before the manipulation is initated: lips parted; mandible lowered slightly from position of closure; tongue in customary, relaxed position; vocal folds not vibrating.

SIMULTANEOUS STIMULATION. Stimulator places fingers in position on respondent's face. As the manipulation takes place, the respondent may observe the stimulator's face and/or hear an auditory stimulus.

EXTRAORAL MANIPULATION /ɑ/ (c**a**lm, l**o**t)

1. Assume starting position.
2. Place thumb and middle finger on mid-chin points 2.
3. Press inward and guide mandible further downward.
4. Phonate after mandible has assumed position.

If the above manipulation is not sufficient, use the additional manipulation procedures.

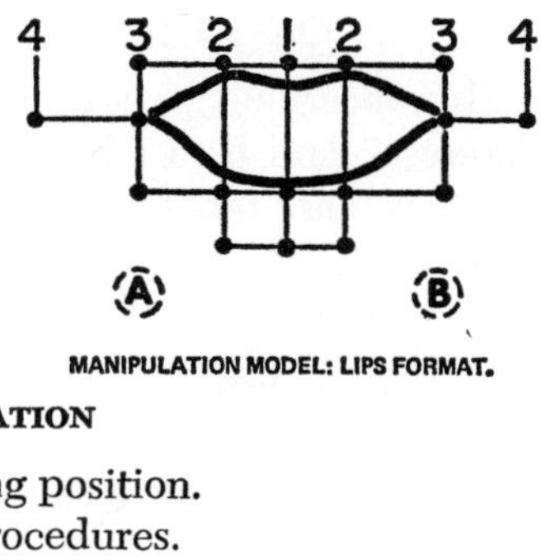

MANIPULATION MODEL: LIPS FORMAT.

ADDITIONAL MANIPULATION

1. Return to starting position.
2. Repeat above procedures.

3. If the head tends to fall forward, use the palm of the opposite hand to push against the respondent's forehead.
4. Phonate. (The stimulator may signal phonation by placing little finger against respondent's larynx.)

/ɑ/ (c*a*lm, l*o*t) Response Analysis and Extraoral Cues

MANDIBLE. If the learner is too tense to allow the mandible to be lowered easily, the stimulator should gently move the respondent's mandible from side-to-side until sufficient relaxation is achieved. If the respondent's head moves forward or downward when the stimulation is applied to the mandible, stabilization may be achieved by the firm placement of the stimulator's hand against the respondent's forehead. If the mandible drops too low and the mouth opening becomes too wide during the stimulation, the little finger of the hand used to stimulate the lower lip may be hooked under the chin to prevent excessive mandibular depression.

LIPS. Rounding of the lips may result in the production of the /ɔ/ (s*aw*, w*a*r). Placing the thumb and middle finger on mid-lip points 3 will help maintain the lips in an unrounded position while lowering the mandible with the other hand.

TONGUE. An undesirable vocal quality may result from a tongue that is too tense, retracted, or too depressed. Elevation of the back of the tongue may cause nasality.

NASAL PORT. If the airstream is being emitted through the nose, the stimulator can place the index finger under the nose of the respondent in order to indicate that the airstream is being improperly emitted. The stimulator should accompany the *tactile* cue with the *visual* cue of shaking his head "no" or *auditory* cue by saying "no."

VOCAL FOLDS. The stimulator's little finger may be placed against the respondent's larynx to signal phonation.

/ɑ/ (c*a*lm, l*o*t) PHONODENTAL GUIDES

Chapter 5 gives details concerning preparation and placement of phonodental guides. Figures 5 and 6 in Chapter 5 illustrate the approximate points of lingual contact for the guides.

Phonodental guides and intraoral cues may be used independently or in combination with the extraoral manipulations.

The extraoral manipulation is usually effective for eliciting *this phoneme, and intraoral stimulation is not required.* If intraoral stimulation is needed, one or more of the following phonodental guides may be utilized.

Stemmed Wire Guides /ɑ/ (c*a*lm, l*o*t)

Lower tongue body: stemmed reflexor used to stimulate body of tongue so it will assume low position by touching tongue tip lightly or by gently drawing reflexor along midline.

Cue Sticks /ɑ/ (c*a*lm, l*o*t)

Cotton-tipped sticks dipped in cold water or parts of tongue depressors may be used to stimulate the same points for lingual contact as those given above.

Note: This sound is easily stimulated and is one of the basic vowels used in syllables and words for stimulating target consonant sounds.

/ɑ/ (c*a*lm, l*o*t) SELECTED PHONEME CHARACTERISTICS

DEVELOPMENTAL AGE:[1]
3 years

FREQUENCY OF OCCURRENCE OF PHONEME:[2]
2.06%, eighteenth in order of occurrence

VISUAL INTELLIGIBILITY:[3]
range—58% to 75%; composite 61%

VISUAL CONFUSION:[4]
/ɑ/ (c*a*lm, /ɚ/ (sist*er*)

AUDITORY INTELLIGIBILITY IN MILD-TO-SEVERE HEARING IMPAIRMENTS:[5]
88%

AUDITORY CONFUSION:[6]
/ei, æ, ɛ, ɑ/ (g*a*te, *a*t, b*e*t, c*a*lm and l*o*t)

RELATIVE PHONETIC POWER:[7]
600 (range of 1 to 680)

PHONEMIC CONFUSION:[8]
/ɑ/ (c*a*lm, l*o*t); /a/ (French l*a*); /ɔ/ (s*aw*, w*a*r)

TYPICAL SPELLING:
a (f*a*ther); *aa* (*aa*rdvark); *al* (p*al*m); *ah* (Ut*ah*); *a* (*r*), (*a*rm); *au* (*au*nt); *e* (*e*ncore); *ea* (h*ea*rt); *ho* (*ho*nor); *on* (*on*); *ow* (kn*ow*ledge); *ua* (g*ua*rd)

/ɑ/ (c*a*lm, l*o*t) PRACTICE MATERIALS

The sound to be stimulated is /ɑ/ (c*a*lm, l*o*t). Only those words and phrases in which the respondent can articulate all of the sounds correctly, except for the target phoneme, should be utilized for practice. The same stipulation applies to the practice materials provided at the end of this Section.

[1-8] *Ibid.* (see p. 79).

/h/ ah, ha, hop, hot; /p/ opera, pa, pop, pot; /b/ obbligato, Bob, bog, bomb; /t/ otter, top, Tod, Tom; /d/ odd, dot, dock, dog; /k/ ox, cop, cot, calm; /g/ Ogg, got, gone, gong; /m/ omelet, mop, mob, mom; /n/ honor, knob, knot, nod; /ŋ/ gong, wrong, tong, long; /hw/ what; /w/ wad, watch, wash, want; /f/ office, fog, father, farm, fob; /v/ Ave Maria, vodka; /ð/ bother; /s/ sob, sod, song, Psalm; /z/ Oz, zombi; /ʃ/ shop, shot, shock; /tʃ/ Cha cha cha, chop, Chang, char; /dʒ/ John, job, jot, jog; /l/ olive, la, log, lock; /r/ arc, are, rob, rock; /j/ yah, yon. *Phrases:* Tom nods. Tom rang the wrong gong. What knob? Bob will watch the shop.

COMPARATIVE PRACTICE MATERIALS

SECTION B: BACK VOWELS

The sounds to be stimulated are /u, ʊ, ɔ, ɑ/ (b*oo*t, f*oo*t, s*a*w and w*a*r, c*a*lm and l*o*t). Only those words and phrases in which the respondent can articulate all of the sounds correctly, except for the target phoneme, should be utilized for practice.

	/u/ (b*oo*t)	/ʊ/ (f*oo*t)	/ɔ/ (s*a*w, w*a*r)	/ɑ/ (c*a*lm, l*o*t)
INITIAL POSITION:	ooze		awes	Oz
MEDIAL POSITION:	pool	pull	Paul	palm
	buhl	book	ball	balm
	cuckoo	cook	caulk	cock
	root		wrought	rot
FINAL POSITION:	moo		maw	ma
	who		haw	ha
	coo		caw	
	you		yaw	
	Lou		law	la

SECTION C: CENTRAL VOWELS

Representative Words:	c*u*p	sof*a*	b*ir*d	sist*er*
International Phonetic Alphabet:	/ʌ/	/ə/	/ɝ/	/ɚ/
Webster's New Collegiate Dictionary (1965):	ˈə	ə	ˈər	ər
Thorndike-Barnhardt Comprehensive				

Dictionary (1951):	u	ə	ėr	ər
Northampton Charts (Yale, 1946):	-u-	-u-	ur	—

Stimulation Units are provided for the central vowels. These include the low back central, lax, unrounded /ʌ/ (c*u*p), mid-central, lax, unrounded /ə/ (sof*a*), mid-central retroflex, tense, half-rounded /ɝ/ (b*ir*d), and mid-central retroflex, lax, half-rounded /ɚ/ (sist*er*).

The central unstressed /ɚ/ (sist*er*) is formed as the /ɝ/ (b*ir*d). There is no acoustic difference between the sounds. The vowel /ɝ/ (b*ir*d) is used in a stressed position such as in b*ir*d; the vowel /ɚ/ is used in an unstressed position as in sist*er*. The tongue obliquely crosses from the occlusional portion of the molars to the gingival portion of the first molars. The tongue apex is curled to a superior retroflex position. The mandible is depressed slightly from the rest position.

The /ɜ/ sound is the nonretroflex equivalent of /ɝ/. The mandible is in the same position as for the /ɝ/. The difference in production is that the tongue apex is not in a retroflex positon, thus the *r*-quality is only slight or absent altogether. It is not necessary to spend time in teaching this sound to a speaker who does not have the nonretroflex sound in his speech area. Concentrate on /ɝ/ (b*ir*d) instead of /ɜ/ (b*ir*d).

The central unstressed /ɚ/ (sist*er*) is formed as the /ɝ/ (b*ir*d). There is little, if any, acoustic difference between the sounds. The vowel /ɝ/ (b*ir*d) is used in a stressed position such as in b*ir*d; the vowel /ɚ/ is used in an unstressed position as in sist*er*.

The same statement can be made for the central vowels /ʌ/ (c*u*p) and /ə/ (sof*a*). The /ʌ/ (c*u*p) is used in a stressed position as in *u*p; the vowel /ə/ is used in unstressed positions such as the last sound in sof*a*.

The unrounded lips play no important role and remain in neutral position. The mandible is depressed to approximately the position of the mid-front vowels.

Stimulation Unit 9

Phonetic Symbol and Representative Word: /ʌ, ə/ (c*u*p, sof*a*)

Symbol Systems

International Phonetic Alphabet: /ʌ/, /ə/
Webster's New Collegiate Dictionary (1965): ˈə, ə

Thorndike-Barnhardt Comprehensive Dictionary (1951): u, ə
Northampton Charts (Yale, 1946): -u-, -u-

Topographical Relationships of Phoneme Production
/ʌ/ (c*u*p) low back central lax unrounded
/ə/ (sof*a*) mid-central lax unrounded

MANDIBLE:
/ʌ/ dropped approximately half as far as /ɑ/
/ə/ approximately the same as /ʌ/ (c*u*p)

LIPS:
/ʌ, ə/ neutral, unrounded, following the position of mandible

TONGUE:
/ʌ, ə/ neutral

AIRSTREAM:
/ʌ, ə/ emitted through mouth

NASAL PORT:
/ʌ, ə/ closed

VOCAL FOLDS:
/ʌ, ə/ vibrating

Stimulation Procedures

VISUAL-AUDITORY MODEL. A model demonstration is provided by the manipulation of the stimulator's face while the respondent observes. An auditory stimulus is usually given simultaneously as the stimulator is saying: "We are going to say /ʌ/ (c*u*p) or /ə/ (sof*a*)." This step may be repeated.

STARTING POSITION. Respondent's articulators should be in the starting position before the manipulation is initiated: lips parted; mandible lowered slightly from position of closure; tongue in customary, relaxed position; vocal folds not vibrating.

SIMULTANEOUS STIMULATION. Stimulator places fingers in position on respondent's face. As the manipulation takes place, the respondent may observe the stimulator's face and/or hear an auditory stimulus.

EXTRAORAL MANIPULATION /ʌ, ə/ (c*u*p, sof*a*)

The /ʌ/ (c*u*p) and /ə/ (sof*a*) are difficult to stimulate, since the lips and tongue are neutral.

1. Assume starting position.
2. Place thumb and middle finger on mid-chin points 2.
3. Shake lower mandible gently, thus relaxing tongue and lips.
4. Phonate. (The stimulator may signal phonation by placing little finger against respondent's larynx.)

5. Provide repetitive auditory samples after each sample until target phoneme is produced.

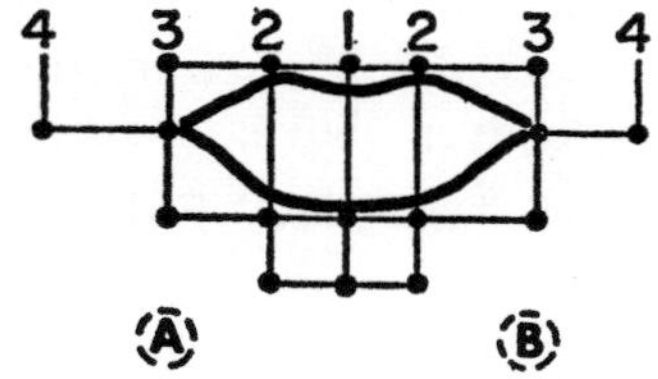

MANIPULATION MODEL: LIPS FORMAT.

/ʌ, ə/ (*cup*, sof*a*) Response Analysis and Extraoral Cues

MANDIBLE. If the respondent is too tense to allow the mandible to be lowered easily, the stimulator should gently move the respondent's mandible from side-to-side until sufficient relaxation is achieved. If the respondent's head moves forward or downward when the stimulation is applied to the mandible, stabilization may be achieved by the firm placement of the stimulator's hand against the respondent's forehead. If the mandible drops too low and the mouth opening becomes too wide during the stimulation, the little finger of the hand used to stimulate the lower lip may be hooked under the chin to prevent excessive mandibular depression.

LIPS AND TONGUE. The lips and tongue are neutral. If the lips become too rounded, the central back sounds are approximated.

NASAL PORT. If the airstream is being emitted through the nose, the stimulator can place the index finger under the nose of the respondent in order to indicate that the airstream is being improperly emitted. The stimulator should accompany the *tactile* cue with the *visual* cue of shaking his head "no" or an *auditory* cue by saying "no."

VOCAL FOLDS. The stimulator's little finger may be placed against the respondent's larynx to signal phonation.

/ʌ, ə/ (*cup*, sof*a*) PHONODENTAL GUIDES

Chapter 5 gives details concerning preparation and placement of phonodental guides. Figures 5 and 6 in Chapter 5 illustrate the approximate points of lingual contact for the guides.

Phonodental guides and intraoral cues may be used independently or in combination with the extraoral manipulations. If intraoral stimulation is needed, one or more of the following phonodental guides may be utilized.

Stemmed Wire Guides /ʌ, ə/ (*cup*, sof*a*)

Lower tongue body: stemmed reflexor used to stimulate body of tongue so it will assume low position by touching tongue tip lightly or by gently drawing reflexor along midline.

Cue Sticks /ʌ, ə/ (c*u*p, sof*a*)

Parts of tongue depressors may be used to stimulate the same points for lingual contact as those given above.

/ʌ, ə/ (c*u*p, sof*a*) SELECTED PHONEME CHARACTERISTICS

DEVELOPMENTAL AGE:[1]

3 years—same for both

FREQUENCY OF OCCURRENCE OF PHONEME:[2]

/ʌ/ 1.32%; thirty-first in order of occurrence

/ə/ 7.26%; third in order of occurrence

VISUAL INTELLIGIBILITY:[3]

/ʌ/ range—27% to 50%; composite 44%

/ə/ range—73% to 100%; composite 79%

VISUAL CONFUSION:[4]

/ɛ, ɪ, ʌ/ (b*e*t, *i*t, c*u*p); /ə/ not given

AUDITORY INTELLIGIBILITY IN MILD-TO-SEVERE HEARING IMPAIRMENTS:[5]

/ʌ/ 83%, /ə/ not given

AUDITORY CONFUSION:[6]

/ɪ, ɛ, ʊ, ʌ, æ/ (*i*t, b*e*t, f*oo*t, c*u*p, *a*t); /ə/ not given

RELATIVE PHONETIC POWER:[7]

/ʌ/ 510; /ə/ not given (range 1 to 680)

PHONEMIC CONFUSION:[8]

/ʌ/ (c*u*p) not given; /ə/ (sof*a*), (b*ir*d—as pronounced by some speakers), /ɪ/ (*i*t), /ʊ/ (f*oo*t)

TYPICAL SPELLING:

/ʌ/ *o* (c*o*ver); *oe* (d*oe*s); *oo* (fl*oo*d); *ou* (tr*ou*ble); *u* (*u*p); /ə/ *a* (sof*a*); *aa* (Is*aa*c); *ah* (pari*ah*); *ai* (fount*ai*n); *e* (mom*e*nt); *eo* (flag*eo*let); *i* (char*i*ty); *ia* (essent*ia*l); *ou* (cauti*ou*s); *o* (c*o*nnect); *u* (*u*pon); *y* (eth*y*l).

/ʌ, ə/ (c*u*p, sof*a*) PRACTICE MATERIALS

The sounds to be stimulated are /ʌ/ (c*u*p) or /ə/ (sof*a*). Only those words and phrases in which the respondent can articulate all of the sounds correctly, except the target phoneme, should be utilized for practice. The same stipulation applies to the comparative practice materials provided at the end of this Section.

/ʌ/ (c*u*p):

/h/ hum, hub, hug, hut; /p/ up, putt, pug, pun; /b/ bum, bug, but,

[1-8] *Ibid.* (see p. 79).

bus; /t/ tub, ton, utmost; /d/ udder, dud, dug, done; /k/ come, cub, cut, cup; /g/ gum, gun, ugly, gushing; /m/ mum, mutt, mass, mother; /n/ numb, nub, nut, nun; /ŋ/ hung, sung, rung, tongue; /w/ won; /f/ fun; /v/ love, glove; /θ/ thumb, thug; /ð/ other, another; /s/ sun, some, us, sub; /z/ buzz; /ʃ/ usher, shut, shuck, shun, /tʃ/ chuck, chubby, touch, Dutch; /dʒ/ judge, just, jump, jug; /l/ ultra, luck, love; /r/ rug, rum, rut, run; /j/ young. *Phrases:* Chuck left the umbrella upstairs. Mother, give me some honey on the bun. Shut the oven.

/ə/ (sof*a*):

/h/ ahead; /p/ apply, Kappa, petunia; /b/ above, ablaze, Cuba, Baloon; /t/ attach, data, quota, attend; /d/ ado, soda, Mandalay; /k/ account, circus, Mecca, hocus; /g/ ago, agree, guffaw, galore; /m/ amaze, mama, amass, Amazon; /n/ another, announce, China, annoy; /hw/ awhile; /w/ away; /f/ affair, sofa, buffalo, emphasis; /v/ avoid, silva, movable, vanilla; /θ/ Athena; /ð/ the; /s/ aside, asleep; /z/ Azores, misery; /ʃ/ ashore, ashamed, ambition; /tʃ/ achieve; /dʒ/ ajar, Jeanette; /l/ aloud, alive, along, aimless; /r/ arouse, camera, parasol, arrive. *Phrases:* Athena announced the affair. The buffalo appeared.

Stimulation Unit 10

Phonetic Symbol and Representative Word: /ɝ/, /ɚ/ (bi*r*d, sist*er*)

Symbol Systems

International Phonetic Alphabet: /ɝ/, /ɚ/
Webster's New Collegiate Dictionary (1965): ˈər, ər
Thorndike-Barnhardt Comprehensive Dictionary (1951): er, ər
Northampton Charts (Yale, 1946): ur

Topographical Relationships of Phoneme Production

/ɝ/ (b*ir*d)	mid-central	retroflex	tense	half rounded
/ɚ/ (sist*er*)	mid-central	retroflex	lax	half rounded

MANDIBLE:
Dropped to lower position than high front or high back vowels

LIPS:
/ɚ/ neutral, similar to opening for /ʌ/ /ɝ/ half rounded

TONGUE:
Tip—points upward and backward in retroflex position
Body—bunched toward front part of hard palate
Sides—in contact with molars

AIRSTREAM:
emitted through mouth
NASAL PORT:
closed
VOCAL FOLDS:
vibrating

Stimulation Procedures

VISUAL-AUDITORY MODEL. A model demonstration is provided by the manipulation of the stimulator's face while the respondent observes. An auditory stimulus is usually given simultaneously as the stimulator is saying: "We are going to say /ɝ/ (b*ir*d) or /ɚ/ (sist*er*)." This step may be repeated.

STARTING POSITION. Respondent's articulators should be in the starting position before the manipulation is initiated: lips parted, mandible lowered slightly from position of closure, tongue in customary, relaxed position, vocal folds not vibrating.

SIMULTANEOUS STIMULATION. Stimulator places fingers in position on respondent's face. As the manipulation takes place, the respondent may observe the stimulator's face and/or hear an auditory stimulus.

EXTRAORAL MANIPULATION /ɝ, ɚ/ (b*ir*d, sist*er*)

1. Assume starting position.
2. Tip head backwards.
3. Place thumb and middle finger of one hand on mid-chin points 2.
4. Hold lips in slightly elongated, narrow opening.
5. Place thumb and middle finger of other hand on upper lip points 3.
6. Phonate.

If the above manipulation is not sufficient, use the additional manipulation procedures.

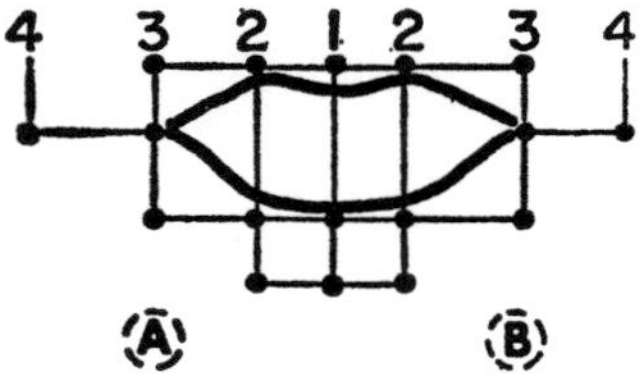

MANIPULATION MODEL: LIPS FORMAT.

ADDITIONAL MANIPULATION

1. Return to starting position.
2. Tip head backwards.

3. Place thumb and middle finger of one hand on mid-chin points 2.
4. Hold lips in slightly elongated, narrow opening.
5. Place thumb and middle finger of other hand on upper lip points 3.
6. Oscillate finger on lip points 3 with short, repetitive movements.
7. Phonate upon each repetitive movement. (The stimulator may signal phonation by placing little finger of the lower hand against respondent's larynx.)

The respondent may tip his head slightly backward while allowing the mandible to drop. This usually encourages the back of the tongue to elevate.

ALTERNATE MANIPULATION

1. Assume starting position.
2. Place thumb and middle finger on upper lip points 3.
3. Hold mandible in slightly lowered position with other hand.
4. Press sides of fingers of other hand under root of tongue (under chin) so tongue "humps up."
5. Phonate. (The stimulator may signal phonation by placing little finger against respondent's larynx.)

/ɝ, ɚ/ (b*ir*d, sist*er*) Response Analysis and Extraoral Cues

LIPS AND TONGUE. The position of the lips and tongue for /ɝ, ɚ/ (b*ir*d, sist*er*) closely approximate those for /ɜ, ə/ as pronounced by some speakers. The /ɝ, ɚ/ (b*ir*d, sist*er*) are used generally, however. No effort should be made to change either pronunciation.

In /ɝ, ɚ/ (b*ir*d, sist*er*) the tongue tip points upward and backward, (retroflex) instead of lying flat, or it may "hump up" toward the front part of the hard palate with the tip down.

NASAL PORT. If the airstream is being emitted through the nose, the stimulator may place the index finger under the nose of the respondent in order to indicate that the airstream is being improperly emitted. The stimulator should accompany the *tactile* cue with the *visual* cue of shaking his head "no" or an *auditory* cue by saying "no."

VOCAL FOLDS. The stimulator's little finger may be placed against the respondent's larynx to signal phonation.

/ɝ, ɚ/ (b*ir*d, sist*er*) PHONODENTAL GUIDES

Chapter 5 gives details concerning preparation and placement of phonodental guides. Figures 5 and 6 in Chapter 5 illustrate the approximate points of lingual contact for the guides.

Phonodental guides and intraoral cues may be used independently or in combination with the extraoral manipulations. If intraoral stimulation is needed, one or more of the following phonodental guides may be utilized.

Denture Guides /ɝ, ɚ/ (b**ir**d, sist**er**)

Raise tongue sides: two denture guides placed in area of Maxillary First Molars (16 and 26).

Dental Floss Guides /ɝ, ɚ/ (b**ir**d, sist**er**)

Raise tongue sides: one stretched dental floss guide placed against crowns of Maxillary First Molars (16 and 26) or slightly posterior; or two knotted dental floss guides between Maxillary First Molars and Second Molars (16-17 and 26-27). Posterior placement of knotted dental floss guides is difficult. Guides may be combined effectively with submandibular pressure.

Stemmed Wire Guides /ɝ, ɚ/ (b**ir**d, sist**er**)

Raise tongue body and tip: forked stemmed wire guide used to push tongue body and tip back and up into approximate areas of Maxillary First Molars (16 and 26).

Cue Sticks /ɝ, ɚ/ (b**ir**d, sist**er**)

A tongue depressor may be used to elevate tongue body and tip.

/ɝ, ɚ/ (b**ir**d, sist**er**) SELECTED PHONEME CHARACTERISTICS

DEVELOPMENTAL AGE:[1]

3 years—same for both

FREQUENCY OF OCCURRENCE OF PHONEME:[2]

/ɝ/ 0.28; thirty-eighth in order of occurrence

/ɚ/ 1.77; twenty-third in order of occurrence

VISUAL INTELLIGIBILITY:[3]

/ɝ/ range—50% to 89%, composite 65%

/ɚ/ range—50% to 89%, composite 65%

VISUAL CONFUSION:[4]

/ɝ/ not given; /ɚ, ɑ/ (sist**er**, c**a**lm and l**o**t)

AUDITORY INTELLIGIBILITY IN MILD-TO-SEVERE HEARING IMPAIRMENTS:[5]

/ɝ/ 80%; /ɚ/ not given

AUDITORY CONFUSION:[6]

not given

RELATIVE PHONETIC POWER:[7]

not given

PHONEMIC CONFUSION:[8]

/ɝ/ (b**ir**d), /r/ (**r**at), /ɜ/ (b**ir**d—as pronounced by some speakers) /ʊ/ (f**oo**t); not given

TYPICAL SPELLING:

/ɝ/ *ear* (*ear*th); *er* (*er*mine); *eur* (entrepren*eur*); *err* (*err*); *ir* (*ir*k); *olo* (c*olo*nel); *or* (w*or*d); *our* (j*our*ney); *ur* (t*ur*n); *yr* (m*yr*tle); /ɚ/ *ar* (pol*ar*ize); *er* (adv*er*tize); *ir* (elix*ir*); *oir* (av*oir*dupois); *or* (arm*or*y); *our* (hon*our*); *re* (ac*re*age); *ur* (aug*ur*); *yr* (zeph*yr*)

/ɝ, ɚ/ (b*ir*d, sist*er*) PRACTICE MATERIALS

The sounds to be stimulated are /ɝ/ (b*ir*d) and /ɚ/ (sist*er*). Only those words and phrases in which the respondent can articulate all of the sounds correctly, except for the target phoneme, should be utilized for practice. The same stipulation applies to the comparative practice materials provided at the end of this Section.

/ɝ/ (b*ir*d)

err; /h/ heard, herds, hurt, Herman; /p/ purr, perk, pert, pearl; /b/ urban, burr, Bert, burn, birth; /t/ turn, term, turf, turkey; /d/ dirt, dearth, dirk; /k/ irk, kirk, Curt, curve, curl; /g/ erg, gird, girl, girth; /m/ Irma, myrrh, murky, Merlin; /n/ urn, nurse; /w/ were, weren't, work; /f/ fur, firm, first; /v/ Irving, verb, avert, divert; /θ/ earth, third, mirth, girth; /s/ sir, sermon, serpent, curse; /z/ curs, hers, furs; /tʃ/ urchin, church, churn, chirp, perch; /dʒ/ journal, adjurn, urge, germ; /l/ earl, learn, hurl, unfurl; /j/ yearn. *Phrases:* You were the first girl. Herman earned a third turn. The nurse returned the urn.

/ɚ/ (sist*er*)

/p/ hopper, popper, tapir, zipper; /b/ barber, harbour, Gerber, rubber, member; /t/ trotter, martyr, booter, motor, brighter; /d/ rider, cider, glider, rudder; /k/ milker, sucker, Tucker, liquer; /g/ anger, stagger, dagger, tiger; /m/ dimmer, glamour, hammer, hummer, timer; /n/ dinner; /f/ differ, zepher, heifer, chauffer; /v/ diver, conniver, driver, paver; /ð/ dither, whither, wither, weather; /s/ dicer, pacer, chaser; /z/ miser, lazer, blazer, Caesar; /ʃ/ crusher, usher, Dasher, Fisher; /tʃ/ searcher, etcher, fracture, lecture; /dʒ/ badger, dodger, Roger, danger, major; /l/ sizzler, angler, bugler, bungler; /j/ lawyer, Moyer, Sawyer. *Phrases.* Search for the badger. The angler took the lawyer to dinner. Roger is a major. At dinner, Tucker explained the danger.

COMPARATIVE PRACTICE MATERIALS

SECTION C: CENTRAL VOWELS

The sounds to be stimulated are /ʌ, ə, ɝ, ɚ/ (*cu*p, sof*a*, b*ir*d, sist*er*).

[1-8] *Ibid.* (see p. 79).

Only those words and phrases in which the respondent can articulate all of the sounds correctly, except the target phoneme, should be utilized for practice.

	/ʌ/ (c*u*p)	/ə/ (sof*a*)	/ɝ/ (b*ir*d)	/ɚ/ (sist*er*)
INITIAL POSITION:		away		
		account		
		affair		
		achieve		
MEDIAL POSITION:	hub		Herb	
	but		Bert	
	cut		curt	
	shut		shirt	
	bud		bird	
	cud		curd	
	gull		girl	
	hull		hurl	
	buck		Burke	
	duck		dirk	
	luck		lurk	
	shuck		shirk	
	tuck		Turk	
FINAL POSITION:		Mama		butter
		Cuba		curter
		China		shutter
		sofa		lurker
				shirker
				Tucker

SECTION D: DIPHTHONGS

Representative Words:	m*i*ce	g*a*te	g*o*	c*ow*	b*oy*	m*u*sic, *you*
International Phonetic Alphabet:	/ɑi/	/ei/	/ou/	/ɑu/	/ɔi/	/iu, ju/
Webster's New Collegiate Dictionary (1965):	ī	ā	ō	au̇	ȯi	yu̇, yü
Thorndike-Barnhardt Comprehensive Dictionary (1951):	ī	ā	ō	ou	oi	ū
Northampton Charts (Yale, 1946):	i-e	a-e	o-e	ou, ow	oi	u-e

A diphthong is composed of two vowel sounds coming together in the same syllable. The sounds are continuous rather than two separate sounds. The articulators glide from one position to the other causing the two sounds to be so closely blended that the ear cannot detect the "valley" or end of the receding glides of the initial vowel or the approaching glide of the second element. For these reasons it is said that the second element ends in the *approximate* position of the second sound.

Many phoneticians consider the diphthong in *mice* to be /ɑi/, others hear /aɪ/; some hear the diphthong in *gate* as /ei/ others hear /eɪ/. These differences in pronunciation are of no consequence, for both are acceptable and are widely used. For purposes of this text, the more extreme sounds are used because they facilitate stimulation and are more easily produced.

Stimulation Unit 11

Phonetic Symbol and Representative Word: /ɑi/ (m*i*ce)

Symbol Systems

International Phonetic Alphabet: /ɑi/
Webster's New Collegiate Dictionary (1965): ī
Thorndike-Barnhardt Comprehensive Dictionary (1951): ī
Northampton Charts (Yale, 1946): i-e

/ɑi/ (m*i*ce) Topographical Relationships of Phoneme Production
/ɑ/ (l*o*t, c*a*lm) First Element of Diphthong—
low back lax unrounded

MANDIBLE:
dropped to lowest position
LIPS:
passive and unrounded, presenting largest opening for any vowel
TONGUE:
neutral position, practically flat on floor of mouth
AIRSTREAM:
emitted through mouth
NASAL PORT:
closed
VOCAL FOLDS:
vibrating

/i/ (b*e*) Second Element of Diphthong—
high front tense unrounded

MANDIBLE:
slightly lowered from position of closure
LIPS:
drawn back in tense position; opening appears as long horizontal line
TONGUE:
Tip—at or near base of lower front teeth
Body—arched and forward
Sides—in contact with upper molars
AIRSTREAM:
emitted through small forward opening between tongue and palate
NASAL PORT:
closed
VOCAL FOLDS:
vibrating

Stimulation Procedures

VISUAL-AUDITORY MODEL. A model demonstration is provided by the manipulation of the stimulator's face while the respondent observes. An auditory stimulus is usually given simultaneously as the stimulator is saying: "We are going to say /ɑi/ (m*i*ce)." This step may be repeated.

STARTING POSITION. Respondent's articulators should be in the starting position before the manipulation is initiated: lips parted; mandible lowered slightly from position of closure; tongue in customary, relaxed position; vocal folds not vibrating.

SIMULTANEOUS STIMULATION. Stimulator places fingers in position on respondent's face. As the manipulation takes place, the respondent may observe the stimulator's face and/or hear an auditory stimulus.

EXTRAORAL MANIPULATION /ɑi/ (m*i*ce)

1. Assume starting position.
2. Place thumb and middle finger of one hand on lower lip points 2.
3. Press inward and guide mandible further downward.
4. Phonate after mandible has assumed position.
5. Continue phonating while pressing inward and sliding fingers into "smile position." (The stimulator may signal phonation by placing little finger against respondent's larynx.)

If the above manipulation is not sufficient, refer to stimulation Units 8 and 1 for the vowel stimulations.

The two elements can be stimulated independently at first, then blended slowly. As the respondent acquires skill in producing the two sounds successively, blending time can be reduced. A sudden movement from the /ɑ/ (c*a*lm, l*o*t) to the /i/ (b*e*) can often achieve a satisfactory blend.

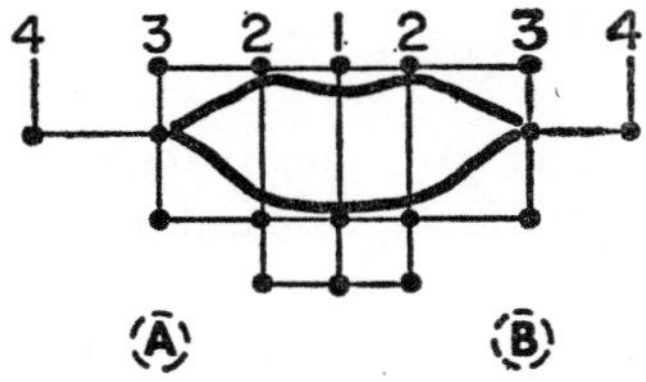

MANIPULATION MODEL: LIPS FORMAT.

/ɑi/ (m*i*ce) Response Analysis and Phonodental Guides

It is assumed that the vowels making up this diphthong were learned before this diphthong is attempted. See Stimulation Units 8 and 1 for details. Figures 5 and 6 in Chapter 5 illustrate the approximate points of lingual contact for the guide.

/ɑi/ (m*i*ce) SELECTED PHONEME CHARACTERISTICS

DEVELOPMENTAL AGE:[1]
3 years

FREQUENCY OF OCCURRENCE OF PHONEME:[2]
2.60%; fourteenth in order of occurrence

VISUAL INTELLIGIBILITY:[3]
range—64% to 75%; composite 64%

VISUAL CONFUSION:[4]
not given

AUDITORY INTELLIGIBILITY IN MILD-TO-SEVERE HEARING IMPAIRMENTS:[5]
79%

AUDITORY CONFUSION:[6]
/ɔi, ɔ, ɑi, æ/ (b*oy*, s*aw* and w*a*r, m*i*ce, *a*t); /ei, ɑi, ɔ/ (g*a*te, m*i*ce, s*aw* and w*a*r)

RELATIVE PHONETIC POWER:[7]
not given

PHONEMIC CONFUSION:[8]
not given

TYPICAL SPELLING:
ai (*ai*sle); *ay* (*ay*); *ei* (h*ei*ght); *eye* (*eye*); *i* (m*i*ce); *ie* (p*ie*); *igh* (h*igh*); *is* (*is*land); *oi* (ch*oi*r); *uy* (g*uy*); *y* (fr*y*); *ye* (d*ye*)

[1-8] *Ibid.* (see p. 79).

/ɑi/ (m*i*ce) PRACTICE MATERIALS

The sound to be stimulated is /ɑi/ (m*i*ce). Only those words and phrases in which the respondent can articulate all of the sounds correctly, except for the target phoneme, should be utilized for practice. The same stipulation applies to the practice materials provided at the end of this Section.

/h/ high, hide, hike, hive; /p/ pie, pike, pies; /b/ buy, bite, bike, bile; /t/ item, tie, time, type; /d/ idea, die, dive, dime; /k/ Ike, kind, kite, Kyle; /g/ guy, guile, guide, guise; /m/ I'm, my, mine, might; /n/ Ina, nigh, deny, nine; /hw/ why?, whine, white, while; /w/ why!, wine, wipe, wide; /f/ Eiffel, fie, fine, fight; /v/ ivy, vie, vine, vice; /θ/ thighed, thighbone; /ð/ either, thy; /s/ ice, sigh, sign, sight; /z/ eyes, Isaiah, design, desire; /ʃ/ shy, shied, shive, shies; /tʃ/ chime, chide, chives, child; /dʒ/ Giles, jive; /l/ island, lie, lime, light; /r/ Ryan, iron, rye, rhyme, ripe; /j/ yipe. *Phrases:* Ryan is fine. Giles was kind to the child. Hide your eyes from the light.

Stimulation Unit 12

Phonetic Symbol and Representative Word: /ei/ (g*a*te)

Symbol Systems

International Phonetic Alphabet: /ei/
Webster's New Collegiate Dictionary (1965): ā
Thorndike-Barnhardt Comprehensive Dictionary (1951): ā
Northampton Charts (Yale, 1946): a-e

/ei/ (g*a*te) Topographical Relationships of Phoneme Production
/e/ (v*a*cation) First Element of Diphthong—mid front
tense unrounded

MANDIBLE:
dropped to a position approximately one third of the way between /i/ (b*e*) and /æ/ (c*a*t)

LIPS:
drawn back in tense position; opening appears as a horizontal line

TONGUE:
Tip—at or near base of lower front teeth
Body—begins to flatten which increases size of reasonating cavity
Sides—in contact with upper molars

AIRSTREAM:
emitted through mouth

Nasal Port:
closed
Vocal Folds:
vibrating

/i/ (b*e*) Second Element of Diphthong–
high front tense unrounded

Mandible:
slightly lowered from position of closure
Lips:
drawn back in tense position; opening appears as long horizontal line
Tongue:
Tip–at or near base of lower front teeth
Body–arched and forward
Sides–in contact with upper molars
Airstream:
emitted through small forward opening between tongue and palate
Nasal Port:
closed
Vocal Folds:
vibrating

Stimulation Procedures

Visual-Auditory Model. A model demonstration is provided by the manipulation of the stimulator's face while the respondent observes. An auditory stimulus is usually given simultaneously as the stimulator is saying: "We are going to say /ei/ (g*a*te)." This step may be repeated.

Starting Position. Respondent's articulators should be in the starting position before the manipulation is initiated: lips parted; mandible lowered slightly from position of closure; tongue in customary, relaxed position; vocal folds not vibrating.

Simultaneous Stimulation. Stimulator places fingers in position on respondent's face. As the manipulation takes place, the respondent may observe the stimulator's face and/or hear an auditory stimulus.

EXTRAORAL MANIPULATION /ei/ (g*a*te)

1. Assume starting position.
2. Place thumb and middle finger on mid-chin points 2.
3. Press inward and guide mandible farther downward, approxi-

mately half-way between the placement for /i/ (b*e*) and /æ/ (c*a*t).

4. Phonate after mandible has assumed position for /e/ (v*a*cation).
5. Continue phonating while pressing inward and sliding fingers simultaneously toward mid-lip points 3—stretching lips into "smile position." (The stimulator may signal phonation by placing little finger against respondent's larynx.)

If the manipulation under point 5 is not sufficient, refer to Stimulation Unit 1 for the /i/ (b*e*) stimulation.

The two elements can be stimulated independently at first, then blended slowly. As the respondent acquires skill in producing the two sounds successively, blending time can be reduced. A sudden movement from the /e/ (v*a*cation) to the /i/ (b*e*) can often achieve a satisfactory blend.

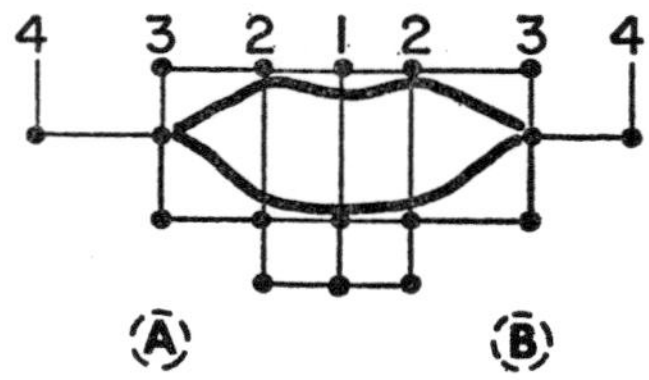

MANIPULATION MODEL: LIPS FORMAT.

/ei/ (v*a*cation) Response Analysis and Extraoral Cues

It is assumed that the vowels making up this diphthong were learned before this diphthong was attempted. See Stimulation Unit 1 for details on the second element of this diphthong.

/e/ (v*a*cation) PHONODENTAL GUIDES

Chapter 5 gives details concerning preparation and placement of phonodental guides. Figures 5 and 6 in Chapter 5 illustrate the approximate points of lingual contact for the guides.

Phonodental guides and intraoral cues may be used independently or in combination with the extraoral manipulations.

The extraoral manipulation is usually effective for eliciting this phoneme, and intraoral stimulation is not required. If intraoral stimulation is needed, one or more of the following phonodental guides may be utilized.

The following describes the use of phonodental guides for the first element /e/ (v*a*cation) of the diphthong. The second element /i/ (b*e*) is described in Stimulation Unit 1. It is assumed that both elements are learned prior to stimulating the diphthong.

Denture Guides /e/ (v*a*cation)

Denture guides are not usually utilized for identifying points of lingual contact for any of the vowels and diphthongs unless other sounds are involved. (See Figure 6.)

Dental Floss Guides /e/ (v*a*cation)

Lower tongue tip: one knotted dental floss guide placed between Mandibular Central Incisors (31-41); or two knotted dental floss guides placed between Mandibular Central Incisors and Lateral Incisors (31-32 and 41-42).

Raise tongue sides: two knotted dental floss guides placed between Maxillary Second Bicuspids and First Molars (15-16 and 25-26).

Stemmed Wire Guides /e/ (v*a*cation)

Lower tongue tip: shorter stem of double-ended wire guide used to position tongue tip behind Mandibular Central Incisors (31-41).

Raise tongue sides: tips of forked stemmed wire guide adjusted so tips touch alveolar ridge in approximate area of Maxillary Second Bicuspids and First Molars (15-16 and 25-26).

Phonodental Guides /i/ (b*e*)

See Stimulation Unit 1.

Cue Sticks /ei/ (g*a*te)

Cotton-tipped sticks dipped in cold water or parts of tongue depressors may be used to stimulate the same points for lingual contact as those given above.

/ei/ (v*a*cation) SELECTED PHONEME CHARACTERISTICS

DEVELOPMENTAL AGE:[1]

3 years

FREQUENCY OF OCCURRENCE OF PHONEME:[2]

/e/ (v*a*cation)—1.94%, twentieth in order of occurrence

VISUAL INTELLIGIBILITY:[3]

range—17% to 75%; composite 48%

VISUAL CONFUSION:[4]

not given

AUDITORY INTELLIGIBILITY IN MILD-TO-SEVERE HEARING IMPAIRMENTS:[5]

100%

AUDITORY CONFUSION:[6]

/ei, ɑi, ɔ/ (g*a*te, m*i*ce, s*aw*)

/ei, æ, ɛ, ɑ/ (g*a*te, *a*t, b*e*t, c*a*lm and l*o*t)

RELATIVE PHONETIC POWER:[7]

370

TYPICAL SPELLING:

a (g*a*te); *ai* (p*ai*n); *ao* (g*ao*l); *ay* (s*ay*); *ea* (gr*ea*t); *ei* (n*ei*ghbor); *et* (chall*et*); *ey* (th*ey*)

/ei/ (v*a*cation) PRACTICE MATERIALS

The sound to be stimulated is /ei/ (g*a*te). Only those words and phrases in which the respondent can articulate all of the sounds correctly, except for the target phoneme, should be utilized for practice. The same stipulation applies to the practice materials provided at the end of this Section.

/h/ hay, hate, hail, haze; /p/ ape, pay, pain, pail; /b/ Abe, bay, bake, baby; /t/ ate, tape, take, tail; /d/ aid, day, date, dame; /k/ ache, Kay, cake, came; /g/ ague, gay, gate, gale; /m/ aim, may, mate, made; /n/ neigh, name, nail, nation; /hw/ whey, whale; /w/ away, wait, wade, wake; /f/ Faye, fate, fade, fame; /v/ Ava, convey, vain, vase; /θ/ atheist, thane; /ð/ they, they'll; /s/ ace, say, safe, same; /z/ *a*'s, Zane, Zahyr; /ʃ/ shay, shape, shade, shake; /ʒ/ Asia, beige; /tʃ/ aitch, chain, change, chafe; /dʒ/ age, James, Jane, jail; /l/ ail, lay, late, lane; /r/ Ray, rate, raid, rake, rain; /j/ yea, Yates, Yale. *Phrases:* Faye caught rain and hail in the pail. Pay James for the race. Ava made a cake.

Stimulation Unit 13

Phonetic Symbol and Representative Word: /ou/ (g*o*)

Symbol Systems

International Phonetic Alphabet: /ou/
Webster's New Collegiate Dictionary (1965): ō
Thorndike-Barnhardt Comprehensive Dictionary (1951): ō
Northampton Charts (Yale, 1946): o-e

/ou/ (g*o*) Topographical Relationships of Phoneme Production
/o/ (*o*bey First Element of Diphthong—
mid back tense rounded

MANDIBLE:

dropped to middle back position—lower than for /u/ (b*oo*t)

LIPS:

rounded and protruded, but less than for /u/ (b*oo*t)

TONGUE:

Tip—Depressed more than for /u/ (b*oo*t)

1-7 *Ibid* (see p. 79).

Body—less elevation and retraction than for /u/ (b*oo*t)
Sides—in contact with Maxillary molars

AIRSTREAM:
emitted through small opening between soft palate and arch of tongue

NASAL PORT:
closed

VOCAL FOLDS:
vibrating

/u/ (b*oo*t) Second Element of Diphthong—
high back tense rounded

MANDIBLE:
at highest position for any back vowel

LIPS:
closely rounded and protruded

TONGUE:
Tip: depressed and retracted
Body: high and back
Sides: in contact with molars

AIRSTREAM:
emitted through small opening between palate and tongue

NASAL PORT:
closed

VOCAL FOLDS:
vibrating

Stimulation Procedures

VISUAL-AUDITORY MODEL. A model demonstration is provided by the manipulation of the stimulator's face while the respondent observes. An auditory stimulus is usually given simultaneously as the stimulator is saying: "We are going to say /ou/ (g*o*)." This step may be repeated.

STARTING POSITION. Respondent's articulators should be in the starting position before the manipulation is initiated: lips parted, mandible lowered slightly from position of closure, tongue in customary, relaxed position, vocal folds not vibrating.

SIMULTANEOUS STIMULATION. Stimulator places fingers in position on respondent's face. As the manipulation takes place, the respondent may observe the stimulator's face and/or hear an auditory stimulus.

EXTRAORAL MANIPULATION /ou/ (g*o*)

1. Assume starting position.
2. Place thumb and middle finger on mid-lip points 3.
3. Direct the corners of the mouth toward mid-lip line 1—forming a rounded opening with protrusion, less than for /u/ (b*oo*t).
4. Phonate.
5. Continue phonating while directing the corners of the mouth farther toward mid-lip line 1—forming a smaller, rounder, and more protruded opening for the second element /u/ (b*oo*t). (The stimulator may signal phonation by placing little finger against respondent's larynx.)

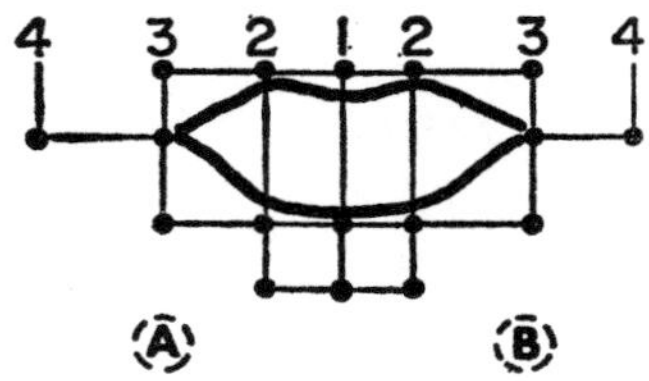

MANIPULATION MODEL: LIPS FORMAT.

/ou/ (g*o*) Response Analysis and Extraoral Cues

It is assumed that the vowels making up this diphthong were learned before this diphthong was attempted. See Stimulation Unit 5 for details related to /u/ (b*oo*t).

/o/ (*o*bey) PHONODENTAL GUIDES

Chapter 5 gives details concerning preparation and placement of phonodental guides. Figures 5 and 6 in Chapter 5 illustrate the approximate points of lingual contact for the guides.

Phonodental guides and intraoral cues may be used independently or in combination with the extraoral manipulations.

The extraoral manipulaton is usually effective for eliciting this phoneme, and *intraoral stimulation is not required.* If intraoral stimulation is needed, one or more of the following phonodental guides may be utilized.

The following describes the use of phonodental guides for the first element /o/ (*o*bey) of the diphthong. The second element /u/ (b*oo*t) is described in Stimulation Unit 5. It is assumed that both elements are learned prior to stimulating the diphthong.

Denture Guides /o/ (*o*bey)

Denture guides are not usually utilized for identifying points of lingual contact, unless other sounds are involved. (See Figure 6.)

Dental Floss Guides /o/ (*o*bey)

Raise tongue sides: two knotted dental floss guides placed between Maxillary First Molars and Second Molars (16-17 and 26-27). The deeper within the oral cavity the knotted dental floss guides must be located, the more difficult they are to place. The use of the forked stemmed guide is recommended.

Stemmed Wire Guides /o/ (*o*bey)

Raise tongue sides: tips of forked stemmed wire guide adjusted so tips touch alveolar ridge in approximate area of Maxillary First Molars and Second Molars (16-17 and 26-27).

Cue Sticks /o/ (*o*bey)

Either cotton-tipped sticks dipped in cold water or parts of tongue depressors may be used to stimulate the same points for lingual contact as those given above.

/ou/ (g*o*) SELECTED PHONEME CHARACTERISTICS

DEVELOPMENTAL AGE:[1]

3 years

FREQUENCY OF OCCURRENCE OF PHONEME:[2]

/o/ (*o*bey)—1.93%; twenty-first in order of occurrence

VISUAL INTELLIGIBILITY:[3]

range—60% to 100%; composite 68%

VISUAL CONFUSION:[4]

not given

AUDITORY INTELLIGIBILITY IN MILD-TO-SEVERE HEARING IMPAIRMENTS:[5]

86%

AUDITORY CONFUSION:[6]

/u, ou/ (b*oo*t, g*o*); /ɑu, ou/ (c*ow*, g*o*); /ou, u, ɔ/ (g*o*, b*oo*t, s*aw*)

RELATIVE PHONETIC POWER:[7]

470

PHONEMIC CONFUSION:[8]

not given

TYPICAL SPELLING:

au (m*au*ve); *eau* (b*eau*); *eo* (y*eo*man); *ew* (s*ew*); *o* (s*o*); *oa* (c*oa*t); *oh* (*oh*); *oe* (t*oe*); *oo* (br*oo*ch); *os* (apropo*s*); *ou* (s*ou*l); *ough* (th*ough*); *ow* (t*ow*); *owe* (*owe*)

/ou/ (g*o*) PRACTICE MATERIALS

The sound to be stimulated is /ou/ (g*o*). Only those words and phrases in which the respondent can articulate all of the sounds cor-

[1-8] *Ibid.* (see p. 79).

rectly, except for the target phoneme, should be utilized for practice. The same stipulation applies to the practice materials provided at the end of this Section.

/h/ oho, hope, home; /p/ open, Poe, poke, pole; /b/ oboe, bow, boat, bore; /t/ oat, toe, tone, toad; /d/ ode, doe, dope, dome; /k/ oak, crow, coat, cone; /g/ ogle, ago, goat, goes; /m/ omen, mow, moat, moan; /n/ own, know, nope, note; /hw/ whoa; /w/ woe, wove, woes; /f/ oaf, foe, folk, phone; /v/ oval, vote; /θ/ oath, throw, thorax; /ð/ though, although, those; /s/ Osler, so, soak, soap; /z/ ozone, zone; /ʃ/ ocean, show, shown, showed; /tʃ/ chore, choke, chose; /dʒ/ Joe, joke, Joan, Joel; /l/ old, low, lobe, loan; /r/ oar, row, rope, robe; /j/ yo-yo, yore, yoke, yeoman. *Phrases:* Does Joe have a phone? Row the boat. Mow the oats.

Stimulation Unit 14

Phonetic Symbol and Representative Word: /ɑu/ (*cow*)

Symbol Systems

International Phonetic Alphabet: /ɑu/
Webster's New Collegiate Dictionary (1965) :aů
Thorndike-Barnhardt Comprehensive Dictionary (1951): ou
Northampton Charts (Yale, 1946): ou, ow

/ɑu/ (*cow*) Topographical Relationships of Phoneme Production
/ɑ/ (*calm, lot*) First Element of Diphthong—
low back lax unrounded

MANDIBLE:
dropped to lowest position
LIPS:
passive and unrounded, presenting largest opening for any vowel
TONGUE:
neutral position, practically flat on floor of mouth
AIRSTREAM:
emitted through mouth
NASAL PORT:
closed
VOCAL FOLDS:
vibrating

/u/ (b*oo*t) Second Element of Diphthong—
high back tense rounded

MANDIBLE:
at highest position for any back vowel
LIPS:
closely rounded and protruded
TONGUE:
Tip—depressed and retracted
Body—high and back
Sides—in contact with molars
AIRSTREAM:
emitted through small opening between palate and tongue
NASAL PORT:
closed
VOCAL FOLDS:
vibrating

Stimulation Procedures

VISUAL-AUDITORY MODEL. A model demonstration is provided by the manipulation of the stimulator's face while the respondent observes. An auditory stimulus is usually given simultaneously as the stimulator is saying: "We are going to say /ɑu/ (c*ow*)." This step may be repeated.

STARTING POSITION. Respondent's articulators should be in the starting position before the manipulation is initiated; lips parted, mandible lowered slightly from position of closure, tongue in customary, relaxed position, vocal folds not vibrating.

SIMULTANEOUS STIMULATION. Stimulator places fingers in position on respondent's face. As the manipulation takes place, the respondent may observe the stimulator's face and/or hear an auditory stimulus.

EXTRAORAL MANIPULATION /ɑu/ (c*ow*)

1. Assume starting position.
2. Place thumb and middle finger on mid-chin points 2.
3. Press inward and guide mandible further downward.
4. Phonate after mandible has assumed position.
5. Continue phonating while placing thumb and middle finger of other hand on mid-lip line 1—forming a small rounded opening. (The stimulator may signal phonation by placing little finger against respondent's larynx.)

If the above manipulation is not sufficient, refer to Stimulation Units 8 and 5.

The two elements can be stimulated independently at first, then blended slowly. As the respondent acquires skill in producing the two sounds successively, blending time can be reduced. A sudden movement from the /ɑ/ (c*a*lm, l*o*t) to the /u/ (b*oo*t) can often achieve a satisfactory blend.

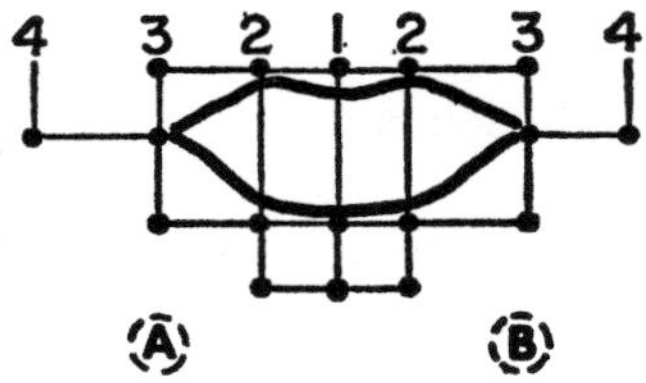

MANIPULATION MODEL: LIPS FORMAT.

/ɑu/ (*cow*) Response Analysis and Phonodental Guides

It is assumed that the vowels making up this diphthong were learned before this diphthong was attempted. See Stimulation Units 8 and 5 for details.

/ɑu/ (*cow*) SELECTED PHONEME CHARACTERISTICS

DEVELOPMENTAL AGE:[1]
3 years

FREQUENCY OF OCCURRENCE OF PHONEME:[2]
0.68%; thirty-fifth in order of occurrence

VISUAL INTELLIGIBILITY:[3]
range—50% to 100%; composite 68%

VISUAL CONFUSION:[4]
not given

AUDITORY INTELLIGIBILITY IN MILD-TO-SEVERE HEARING IMPAIRMENTS:[5]
83%

AUDITORY CONFUSION:[6]
/ɑu, ou/ (c*ow*, g*o*)

RELATIVE PHONETIC POWER:[7]
not given

PHONEMIC CONFUSION:[8]
not given

TYPICAL SPELLING:
au (kr*au*t); *hou* (*hou*r); *ou* (*ou*t) *ough* (b*ough*), *ow* (h*ow*)

[1-8] *Ibid.* (see p. 79).

/ɑu/ (*cow*) PRACTICE MATERIALS

The sound to be stimulated is /ɑu/ (*cow*). Only those words and phrases in which the respondent can articulate all of the sounds correctly, except for the target phoneme, should be utilized for practice. The same stipulation applies to the practice materials provided at the end of this Section.

/h/ how, house, howl, hound; /p/ pout, pouch, pound; /b/ bout, bower, about, bow; /t/ out, outlaw, outside, outfit; /d/ endow, down, douse, dour; /k/ cow, couch, cowl, cowed; /g/ Gow, gout, gown, gouge; /m/ mow, mouse, mouth; /n/ ounce, now, noun; /w/ ow, wow!, wowed, wound; /f/ fowl, found, flower; /v/ vow, avow, vouch, vowel; /θ/ thousand; /ð/ thou; /s/ sow, souse, sour, south; /ʃ/ shout, shower; /tʃ/ ouch, chow; /l/ owl, allow, loud, louse; /r/ our, rout, round, around; /j/ yowl. *Phrases:* Shout out loud. The owl was not allowed around the house. A thousand flowers showered petals on the ground.

Stimulation Unit 15

Phonetic Symbol and Representative Word: /ɔi/ (b*oy*)

Symbol Systems

International Phonetic Alphabet: /ɔi/
Webster's New Collegiate Dictionary (1965): ȯi
Thorndike-Barnhardt Comprehensive Dictionary (1951): oi
Northampton Charts (Yale, 1946): oi

/ɔi/ (b*oy*) Topographical Relationships of Phoneme Production
/ɔ/ (*saw, war*) First Element of Diphthong—low back lax rounded

MANDIBLE:
slightly lower than for /ʊ/ (f*oo*t) sound

LIPS:
open, slightly rounded, but without protrusion

TONGUE:
Tip—near base of lower front teeth
Body—arched upward and backward toward velum
Sides—complete separation from the teeth

AIRSTREAM:
emitted through opening between tongue and palate

NASAL PORT:
closed

VOCAL FOLDS:
vibrating

/i/ (b*e*) Second Element of Diphthong—high front tense unrounded

MANDIBLE:
slightly lowered from position of closure

LIPS:
drawn back in tense position; opening appears as long horizontal line

TONGUE:
Tip—at or near base of lower front teeth
Body—arched and forward
Sides—in contact with upper molars

AIRSTREAM:
emitted through small forward opening between tongue and palate

NASAL PORT:
closed

VOCAL FOLDS:
vibrating

Stimulation Procedures

VISUAL-AUDITORY MODEL. A model demononstration is provided by the manipulation of the stimulator's face while the respondent observes. An auditory stimulus is usually given simultaneously as the stimulator is saying: "We are going to say /ɔi/ (b*oy*)."

STARTING POSITION. Respondent's articulators should be in the starting position before the manipulation is initiated: lips parted; mandible lowered slightly from position of closure; tongue in customary, relaxed position; vocal folds not vibrating.

SIMULTANEOUS STIMULATION. Stimulator places fingers in position on respondent's face. As the manipulation takes place, the respondent may observe the stimulator's face and/or hear an auditory stimulus.

EXTRAORAL MANIPULATION /ɔi/ (b*oy*)

1. Assume starting position.
2. Place thumb and middle finger of one hand on mid-lip points 3.
3. Shape lips into slightly oval form.
4. Place thumb and middle finger of other hand on lower lip points 2.
5. Shape lips into slightly oval form with the upper hand.
6. Phonate after lips have assumed position.
7. Continue phonating while releasing fingers of upper hand.
8. Press inward and slide fingers of lower hand simultaneously

toward mid-lip points 3—stretching lips into "smile position." (The stimulator may signal phonation by placing little finger against respondent's larynx.)

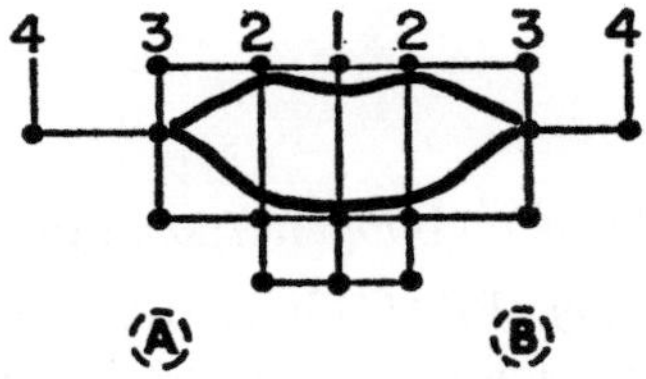

MANIPULATION MODEL: LIPS FORMAT.

If the above stimulation is not sufficient, refer to Stimulation Units 7 and 1 for the stimulations of the single phonemes.

The two elements can be stimulated independently at first, then blended slowly. As the respondent acquires skill in producing the two sounds successively, blending time can be reduced. A sudden movement from /ɔ/ (s*aw*) to /i/ (b*e*) can often achieve a satisfactory blend.

Note: The procedure for the /ɔ/ (s*aw*, w*ar*) may be reversed so that the /ɑ/ (c*a*lm, l*o*t) is stimulated and the shaping of the lips takes place while the /ɑ/ (c*a*lm, l*o*t) is being produced. In the diphthong /ɔi/ (b*oy*), the /ɑ/ (c*a*lm, l*o*t) can be used as a starter with the oval molding for the /ɔ/ (w*ar*, s*aw*) taking place as the extraoral manipulations take the lips into the /i/ (b*e*) position.

/ɔi/ (b*oy*) Response Analysis and Phonodental Guides

It is assumed that the vowels making up this diphthong were learned before this diphthong was attempted. See Stimulation Units 7 and 1 for details.

/ɔi/ (b*oy*) SELECTED PHONEME CHARACTERISTICS

DEVELOPMENTAL AGE:[1]
3 years

FREQUENCY OF OCCURRENCE OF PHONEME:[2]
0.06%; forty-first in order of occurrence

VISUAL INTELLIGIBILITY:[3]
range—66% to 100%; composite 72%

VISUAL CONFUSION:[4]
not given

AUDITORY INTELLIGIBILITY IN MILD-TO-SEVERE HEARING IMPAIRMENTS:[5]
83%

AUDITORY CONFUSION:[6]

/ɔi, ɔ, ɑi, æ/ (b*oy*, s*aw*, m*i*ce, *a*t)

RELATIVE PHONETIC POWER:[7]

not given

PHONEMIC CONFUSION:[8]

not given

TYPICAL SPELLING:

oi (*oi*l); *oy* (r*oy*al); *uoy* (b*uoy*ant); *ois* (Illin*ois*)

/ɔi/ (b*oy*) PRACTICE MATERIALS

The sound to be stimulated is /ɔi/ (b*oy*). Only those words and phrases in which the respondent can articulate all of the sounds correctly, except for the target phoneme, should be utilized for practice. The same stipulation applies to the practice materials provided at the end of this Section.

/ɔi/ oil; /h/ Hoyle, ahoy; /p/ poi, poison, poise; /b/ boy, boil, Boyd; /t/ toy, toil; /d/ Doyle; /k/ coy, coil, coin; /g/ gargoyle; /m/ moil; /n/ ointment, annoy, noise; /f/ Foy, foil; /v/ void, voile, envoy; /s/ oyster, soy, soil, Savoy; /z/ noise, boys; /tʃ/ choice; /dʒ/ Joyce, joy; /l/ oil, Lloyd, loin; /r/ Roy, royal, Royce. *Phrases:* The noise annoys the boys. Boil the oysters.

Stimulation Unit 16

Phonetic Symbol and Representative Word: /iu, ju/ (m*u*sic, *you*)

Symbol Systems

International Phonetic Alphabet: /iu, ju/
Webster's New Collegiate Dictionary (1965): yů, yü
Thorndike-Barnhardt Comprehensive Dictionary (1951): ū
Northampton Charts (Yale, 1946): u-e

/iu, ju/ (m*u*sic, *you*) Topographical Relationships of Phoneme Production

/i/ (b*e*) First Element of Diphthong—high front tense unrounded	/j/ (*y*et) Semidiphthongal linguapalatal glide
MANDIBLE:	
slightly lowered from position of closure	slightly lowered

[1-8] *Ibid.* (see p. 79).

LIPS:		
	drawn back in tense position; opening appears as long horizontal line	neutral position
TONGUE:		
	Tip—at or near base of lower front teeth	at or near base of lower front teeth
	Body—arched and forward	arched and forward
	Sides—in contact with upper molars	in contact with upper molars
AIRSTREAM:		
	emitted through small forward opening between tongue and palate	emitted through narrow opening between tongue and palate as tongue is dropped
NASAL PORT:		
	closed	closed
VOCAL FOLDS:		
	vibrating	vibrating

/u/ (b*oo*t) Topographical Relationships of Phoneme Production
Second Element of Diphthong—high back tense rounded

MANDIBLE:
at highest position for any back vowel

LIPS:
closely rounded and protruded

TONGUE:
Tip—depressed and retracted
Body—high and back
Sides—in contact with molars

AIRSTREAM:
emitted through small opening between palate and tongue

NASAL PORT:
closed

VOCAL FOLDS:
vibrating

Stimulation Procedures

VISUAL-AUDITORY MODEL. A model demonstration is provided by the manipulation of the stimulator's face while the respondent observes. An auditory stimulus is usually given simultaneously with the stimulator saying: "We are going to say /iu, ju/ (m*u*sic, *you*)."

STARTING POSITION. Respondent's articulators should be in the starting position before the manipulation is initiated: lips parted, mandible lowered slightly from position of closure, tongue in customary, relaxed position, vocal folds not vibrating.

SIMULTANEOUS STIMULATION. Stimulator places fingers in position on respondent's face. As the manipulation takes place, the respondent may observe the stimulator's face and/or hear an auditory stimulus.

EXTRAORAL MANIPULATION /iu, ju/ (m*u*sic, *you*)

1. Assume starting position.
2. Place thumb and middle finger of one hand on lower lip points 2.
3. Press inward and slide fingers simultaneously toward mid-lip points 3—stretching lips into "smile position."
4. Begin phonating as lips approximate "smile position."
5. Continue phonating as thumb and middle finger of the other hand are placed at upper lip points 3.
6. Use both hands to direct mouth toward mid-lip line 1—forming a small rounded opening. (The stimulator may signal phonation by placing little finger against the respondent's larynx.)

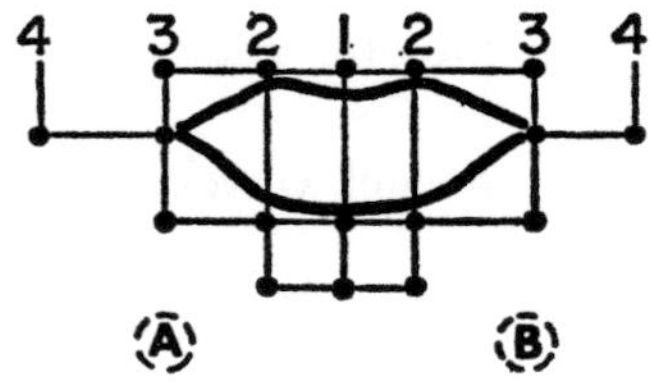

MANIPULATION MODEL: LIPS FORMAT.

If the above manipulation is not sufficient, refer to Stimulation Units 1 /i/ (b*e*) or 39 /j/ (*y*et) and 5 /u/ (b*oo*t).

The two elements can be stimulated independently at first, then blended slowly. As the respondent acquires skill in producing the sounds successively, blending time can be reduced. An *extremely sudden* movement from the first element /j/ (*y*et) to the second element /u/ (b*oo*t) will produce a well defined /j/ (*y*et), thus producing /ju/ (*you*).

Note: The semi-diphthong /ju/ (*you*) and the diphthong /iu/ (m*u*sic) differ only slightly. /j/ (*you*) is usually found in the initial position of a word, following /k/ (*c*ute) and sometimes following /g/ (a*gue*). The acoustical difference is only slight. There is no sematic difference, consequently no issue should be made in distinguishing between the sounds.

/iu, ju/ (m*u*sic, *you*) Response Analysis and Phonodental Guides

It is assumed that the vowels making up this diphthong were learned before the diphthong was attempted.

See Stimulation Units 1, 5 and 32 for details.

/iu, ju/ (m*u*sic, *you*) SELECTED PHONEME CHARACTERISTICS

DEVELOPMENTAL AGE:[1]

3 years

FREQUENCY OF OCCURRENCE OF PHONEME:[2]

not given

VISUAL INTELLIGIBILITY:[3]

not given

VISUAL CONFUSION:[4]

not given

AUDITORY INTELLIGIBILITY IN MILD-TO-SEVERE HEARING IMPAIRMENTS:[5]

not given

AUDITORY CONFUSION:[6]

not given

RELATIVE PHONETIC POWER:[7]

not given

PHONEMIC CONFUSION:[8]

not given

TYPICAL SPELLING:

*ea*u (b*eau*ty); *eu* (f*eu*d); *eue* (Q*ueue*); *ew* (f*ew*); *ewe* (*ewe*); *ieu* (ad*ieu*); *iew* (v*iew*); *u* (m*u*le); *ugh* (H*ugh*); *ue* (c*ue*); *yew* (*yew*); *you* (*you*), *yu* (*yu*le)

/iu, ju/ (m*u*sic, *you*) PRACTICE MATERIALS

The sound to be stimulated is /iu/ (m*u*sic) or /ju/ (*you*). Only those words and phrases in which the respondent can articulate all of the sounds correctly, except for the target phoneme, should be utilized for practice. The same stipulation applies to the practice materials provided at the end of this Section.

/ju/ you; /h/ Hugh, Hume, human, humor; /p/ pew, pure, pews; /b/ imbue, butte, beauty, Beulah; /t/ Ute, virtue, tune, Tuesday; /d/ you'd, adieu, dune; /k/ uke, clue, cube, cute, cues; /g/ ague; /m/ mew, mule, muse, music; /n/ unit, union, new, avenue; /hw/ whew; /f/ few, fuse, feud, fume; /v/ you've, view, viewed; /θ/ youth; /s/ usurp; /z/ use, uses, used; /ʃ/ shoe; /ʒ/ usually; /dʒ/ Jew; /l/

[1-8] *Ibid.* (see p. 79).

you'll, value, lieu; /r/ your. *Phrases:* Beulah flew to Europe. Few refuse you. Review the cues.

COMPARATIVE PRACTICE MATERIALS

SECTION D: DIPHTHONGS

The sounds to be stimulated are /ɑi, ei, ou, ɑu, ɔi, iu, ju/ (m*i*ce, g*a*te, g*o*, c*ow*, b*oy*, m*u*sic, *you*). Only those words and phrases in which the respondent can articulate all of the sounds correctly, except for the target phoneme, should be utilized for practice.

	/ɑi/ (m*i*ce)	/ei/ (g*a*te)	/ou/ (g*o*)	/ɑu/ (c*ow*)	/ɔi/ (b*oy*)	/iu, ju/ (m*u*sic, *you*)
Initial Position:	ice	ace	Oster	ouster	oyster	use
			oat	out	oil	ute
Medial Position:	bite	bait	boat	bout	Boise	Butte
	bile	bail	bowl	bowel	boil	Beulah
	kite	Kate	coat	cowed	coil	cute
	kine	cane	cone	Cowan	coin	Kuhne
	file	fail	foal	fowl	foil	fuel
	fine	feign	phone	found	coif	funeral
	Heil!	hail	hole	howl	Hoyle	Hewlett
	pies	pays	pose	pout	poise	pews
	mice	mace	most	mouse	moist	music
Final Position:	my	may	mow	mau	Quemoy	miew
	pie	pay	Poe	pow	poi	Pugh
	buy	bay	bow	bow	boy	imbue
	die	day	dough	Dow		dew
	high	hay	hoe	how	Hoy	Hugh

SECTIONS FOR CONSONANTS

Introduction

The Sections are divided into nasals, stops, fricatives, sibilants, affricates, semivowels, and a lateral. The English consonant sounds differ from the vowel sounds in that a greater modification of the oral cavity is sometimes required. This modification sometimes results in a certain amount of friction. The durational value of the consonants is that of a stop such as /t/ (*t*o) which is exploded and finished, or of

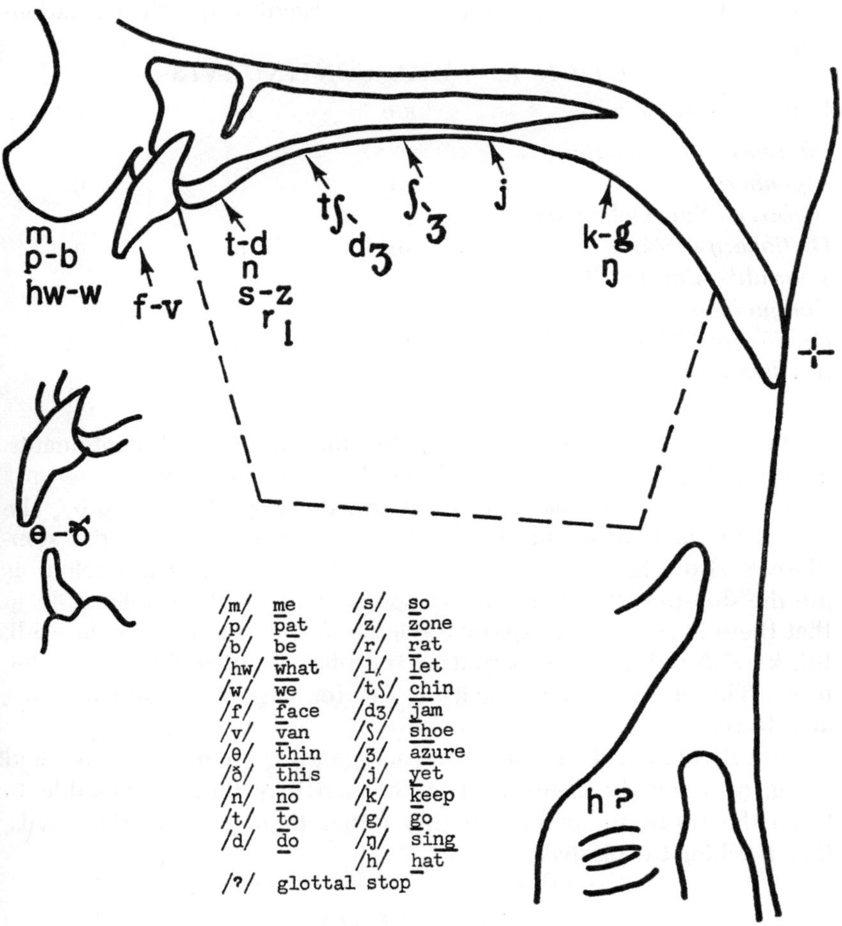

+Nasopharyngeal port open for /m,n, ŋ/.

Figure 11. Placement of consonants.

a continuant such as /n/ (*no*) which can be continued as long as the breath lasts.

Many of the consonants are classified in voiced and voiceless pairs, sometimes called homorganic pairs. The members of the pairs are identical in formation with the exception that the vocal folds vibrate on one member of the pair which results in a voiced sound, and do not vibrate on the other member which results in a voiceless sound.

Figure 11 shows the consonant sounds of English and their relationships.

SECTION E: NASAL CONTINUANTS

Representative Words:	*m*e	*n*o	si*ng*
International Phonetic Alphabet:	m	n	ŋ
Webster's New Collegiate Dictionary (1965):	m	n	ŋ
Thorndike-Barnhardt Comprehensive Dictionary (1951):	m	n	ng
Northampton Charts (Yale, 1946):	m	n	ng

Stimulation Units are provided for the three nasal continuants. The sounds /m, n, ŋ/ are voiced, nasal, continuant sounds. The /m/ sound is blocked by the two lips as are the stop-plosives /p-b/, the /n/ is blocked by tongue tip at the alveolar ridge as are the stop-plosives /t-d/; the /ŋ/ is blocked by back of tongue at the velum as are the stop-plosives /k-g/. These points of articulation differ only in that there is no sudden explosive release in the /m, n, ŋ/ as in /p-b, t-d, k-g/. Nasal emission permits a full pharyngeal resonance on /m, n, ŋ/. The oral resonating cavity is full for /m/, decreased for /n/, and decreased to a greater extent for /ŋ/.

The articulation of the sounds in each group /p, b, m/, /t, d, n/, and /k, g, ŋ/ is nearly identical. The clinician may find it profitable to teach the triplicate sounds together rather than teaching the nasals, then teaching the plosives.

Stimulation Unit 17

Phonetic Symbol and Representative Word: /m/ (*m*e)

Symbol Systems

International Phonetic Alphabet: /m/ (*m*e)
Webster's New Collegiate Dictionary (1965): m
Thorndike-Barnhardt Comprehensive Dictionary (1951): m
Northampton Charts (Yale, 1946): m

Topographical Relationships of Phoneme Production
/m/ (*m*e) voiced bilabial nasal continuant

MANDIBLE:
slightly lowered

LIPS:
closed position
TONGUE:
neutral position
AIRSTREAM:
emitted through nasal passages
NASAL PORT:
open
VOCAL FOLDS:
vibrating

Stimulation Procedures

VISUAL-AUDITORY MODEL. A model demonstration is provided by the manipulation of the stimulator's face while the respondent observes. An auditory stimulus is usually given simultaneously as the stimulator is saying: "We are going to say /m/ (*m*e)." This step may be repeated.

STARTING POSITION. Respondent's articulators should be in the starting position before the manipulation is initiated: lips parted, mandible lowered slightly from position of closure, tongue in customary, relaxed position, vocal folds not vibrating.

SIMULTANEOUS STIMULATION. Stimulator places fingers in position on respondent's face. As the manipulation takes place, the respondent may observe the stimulator's face and/or hear an auditory stimulus.

EXTRAORAL MANIPULATION /m/ (*m*e)

1. Assume starting position.
2. Place thumb and middle finger of one hand on lower lip points 2.
3. Move lower lip toward mid-lip line.
4. Place index finger of other hand gently on side of nose as a signal for nasal resonance.
5. Phonate.

If the above manipulation is not sufficient, use the additional manipulation procedures.

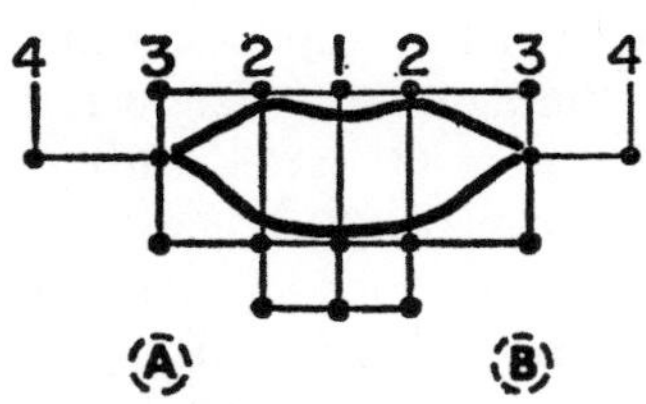

MANIPULATION MODEL: LIPS FORMAT.

ADDITIONAL MANIPULATION

1. Return to starting position.
2. Place thumb and middle finger of one hand on lower lip points 2.
3. Place thumb and middle finger of other hand on upper lip points 2.
4. Move both lips toward mid-lip line.
5. With finger of upper hand, touch side of nose gently as a signal for nasal emission of air.
6. Phonate. (The stimulator may signal phonation by placing little finger against respondent's larynx.)

Adding /ɑ/ (l*o*t, c*a*lm) to /m/ (*m*e) produces an easy syllable for initial practice of the manipulation procedures. A schwa /ə/ (sof*a*) may be heard with a rapid series of /m/ (*m*e).

/m/ (*m*e) Response Analysis and Extraoral Cues

Lips. In production of the /m/ (*m*e), a build-up of air pressure such as that needed for the /p/ (*p*at) and /b/ (*b*e) is not needed, therefore, lip control should be light. Tense lips may produce a /b/ (*b*e) when lips separate. Blowing or trilling lips may help reduce lip tension. The upper lip should not be pulled down.

The finger of the respondent may be placed between the lips of the stimulator to detect the various degrees of pressure and to identify the one that is appropriate for the /p/ (*p*at), /b/ (*b*e), and /m/ (*m*e) sounds.

If the pressure is too great, it may cause a /p/ (*p*at) or /b/ (*b*e) to be added after the /m/ as in /mbi/. A schwa /ə/ (sof*a*) may be added when the /m/ is final as in /hæmə/ for *ham*.

Cheeks. The cheeks should not be puffed out in the production of /m/ (*m*e), /p/ (*p*at), or /b/ (*b*e). Pressing a thumb and finger against the cheeks can reduce puffing.

Airstream. A feather or small strip of paper may be held in front of respondent's or stimulator's lips to compare the degree of explosiveness of /p/ (*p*at), /b/ (*b*e), and /m/ (*m*e).

Nasal Port. Closure or obstruction of the nasal port can cause denasal quality. A finger of the respondent may be placed against his nose and that of the stimulator in order to feel the resonance change when the /m/ (*m*e) sound is alternated with /p/ (*p*at) and /b/ (*b*e).

A mirror may be placed beneath the nostrils of the respondent and/or stimulator to illustrate the moisture caused by the nasal emission of the /m/ (*m*e) in contrast with the /p/ (*p*at) and /b/ (*b*e) sounds.

Vocal Folds. Continued voicing after the articulators assume a different position will cause a vowel or other sound to be added to the /m/ (*me*). The problem is common in the speech of many deaf persons.

Touching the respondent's larynx with a finger can serve as a signal for phonation.

/m/ (*me*) SELECTED PHONEME CHARACTERISTICS

DEVELOPMENTAL AGE:[1]

m-, -m-, -m = 3 yrs.; -mp, -rm, -mr, -sm = 3.5 yrs; sm-, -mpt, -mps = 4 yrs.; -mbr = 5 yrs.; -zm = 7 yrs.

(not reported: md, lm, rmd, mz.)

FREQUENCY OF OCCURRENCE OF PHONEME:[2]

3.16%; tenth in order of occurrence

VISUAL INTELLIGIBILITY:[3]

34%–100%; composite 66%

VISUAL CONFUSION:[4]

/p, b, m/ (*p*at, *b*e, *m*e)

AUDITORY INTELLIGIBILITY IN MILD-TO-SEVERE HEARING IMPAIRMENTS:[5]

78%

AUDITORY CONFUSION:[6]

/m, n, ŋ/ (*m*e, *n*o, si*ng*)

RELATIVE PHONETIC POWER:[7]

52 (range of 1 to 680)

PHONEMIC CONFUSION:[8]

/m/ (*m*e); /b/ (*b*e)

TYPICAL SPELLING:

chm dra*chm*); *gm* (diaphra*gm*); *lm* (pa*lm*); *m* (*m*en); *mb* (co*mb*); *me* (ho*me*); *mm* (ma*mm*a)

/m/ (*me*) PRACTICE MATERIALS

The sound to be stimulated is /m/ (*me*). Only those words and phrases in which the respondent can articulate all of the sounds correctly, except the target phoneme, should be utilized for practice. The same stipulation applies to the comparative practice materials at the end of this Section.

The vowels and diphthongs for use with the target phoneme are arranged with the most easily stimulated first. This arrangement is compatible with the recommendations given in Chapter 6.

/ɑ/ mop, Tom, palm, mama; /u/ moo, moon, room, whomever; /i/ meat, beam, seem, Mimi; /ɑu/ mouth, mouse, mountain, Baum; /ɑi/

[1-8] *Ibid.* (see p. 79).

my, mine, time, chimes; /ju/ mule, mute, fume, amuse; /ou/ Moe, comb, home, foaming; /ei/ May, name, same, James; /ɑu/ mound, mouth, mouse; /ɪ/ mitt, miss, him, amiss; /ɛ/ Mel, gem, helmet, lemon; /æ/ map, mass, am, mammy; /ʊ/ moor; /ʌ/ mum, much, thumb, sometime; /ə/ Christmas; /ɝ/ myrrh, mirth, term, German; /ɚ/ homer, timer, firmer. *Phrases:* Many men marry at Christmas. Pam missed Meg at the game. Maude's remarks amazed my mother.

Stimulation Unit 18

Phonetic Symbol and Representative Word; /n/ (*n*o)

Symbol Systems

International Phonetic Alphabet: /n/
Webster's New Collegiate Dictionary (1965): n
Thorndike-Barnhardt Comprehensive Dictionary (1951): n
Northampton Charts (Yale, 1946): n

Topographical Relationships of Phoneme Production
/n/ (*n*o) voiced lingua-alveolar nasal continuant

MANDIBLE:
slightly lowered
LIPS:
slightly open to follow line of depression of mandible
TONGUE:
Tip—raised to make contact with alveolar ridge back of upper front teeth
Sides—in contact with upper teeth
AIRSTREAM:
emitted through nasal passages
NASAL PORT:
open
VOCAL FOLDS:
vibrating

Stimulation Procedures

VISUAL-AUDITORY MODEL. A model demonstration is provided by the manipulation of the stimulator's face while the respondent observes. An auditory stimulus is usually given simultaneously as the stimulator is saying: "We are going to say /n/ (*n*o)." This step may be repeated.

STARTING POSITION. Respondent's articulators should be in the starting position before the manipulation is initiated: lips parted, mandible lowered slightly from position of closure, tongue in customary, relaxed position, vocal folds not vibrating.

SIMULTANEOUS STIMULATION. Stimulator places fingers in position on respondent's face. As the manipulation takes place, the respondent may observe the stimulator's face and/or hear an auditory stimulus.

EXTRAORAL MANIPULATION /n/ (*no*)

1. Assume starting position.
2. Place side of middle finger of one hand along upper lip line between points 2.
3. Place index finger of other hand, or same hand, gently on side of nose as a signal for nasal resonance.
4. Phonate.

If the above manipulation is not sufficient, use the additional manipulation procedures.

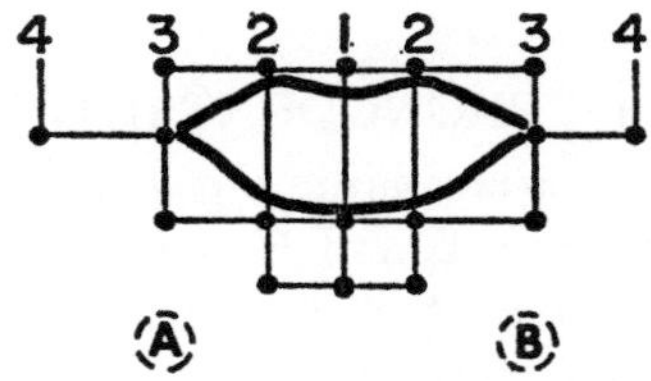

MANIPULATION MODEL: LIPS FORMAT.

ADDITIONAL MANIPULATION

1. Return to starting position.
2. Place side of middle finger of one hand along upper lip line between points 2.
3. Place index finger of same hand gently on side of nose as a signal for nasal emission of air.
4. If needed, use little finger of other hand to lower mandible slightly.
5. Use thumb and third finger of second hand near lip line 3 and move lips slightly outward.
6. Phonate. (The stimulator may signal phonation by placing a finger of the lower hand against respondent's larynx.)

Adding /ɑ/ (l*o*t, c*a*lm) to /n/ (*n*o) produces an easy syllable for initial practice of the manipulation procedures.

/n/ (*no*) Response Analysis and Extraoral Cues

MANDIBLE. The mandible may be dropped inappropriately for the

/n, t, d/ (*no*, *to*, *do*) when these sounds are produced with the tongue tip down and the forward part of the tongue body obstructs the air by pressing against the alveolar ridge.

TONGUE. When the tip of the tongue is placed behind the lower incisors, the lingual contact with the upper incisors is made with the body of the tongue.

If the tongue tip is withdrawn suddenly after a final /n/ (*no*), a /t/ (*to*) or /d/ (*do*) may be audible as in /mænt, mænd/ for *man.*

NASAL PORT. A finger of the respondent may be placed against the nose of the respondent and of the stimulator so that the change in resonance can be felt when the /n/ (*no*) sound is alternated with /t/ (*to*) and /d/ (*do*).

Closure or obstruction of the nasal port can cause denasal quality.

VOCAL FOLDS. Continued voicing of the /n/ (*no*) after the articulators assume a different position will cause a vowel or other sound to be added to the /n/ (*no*), for example, /fʌnə/ for *fun.*

Touching the respondent's larynx with a finger can serve as a signal for phonation.

/n/ (*no*) PHONODENTAL GUIDES

Chapter 5 gives details concerning preparation and placement of phonodental guides. Figures 5 and 6 in Chapter 5 illustrate the approximate points of lingual contact for the guides.

Phonodental guides and intraoral cues may be used independently or in combination with the extraoral manipulations.

The extraoral manipulation is usually effective for eliciting this phoneme, and intraoral stimulation is not required. If intraoral stimulation is needed, one or more of the following phonodental guides may be utilized.

Denture Guides /n/ (*no*)

Raise tongue tip: one guide is placed between Maxillary Central Incisors (11-21).

Dental Floss Guides /n/ (*no*)

Raise tongue tip: one knotted dental floss guide placed between Maxillary Central Incisors (11-21).

Stemmed Wire Guides /n/ (*no*)

Raise tongue tip: longer stem of double-ended wire guide used to position tongue tip behind Maxillary Central Incisors (11-21).

Cue Sticks /n/ (*no*)

Cotton-tipped sticks dipped in cold water or parts of tongue depressors may be used to stimulate the same points for lingual contact as those given above.

/n/ (*no*) SELECTED PHONEME CHARACTERISTICS

DEVELOPMENTAL AGE:[1]

n-, -n-, -n = 3 yrs.; -nr = 3.5 yrs.; sn- = 4 yrs.; -rn = 5 yrs.; -nt, -nd, -ntth = 6 yrs.

FREQUENCY OF OCCURRENCE OF PHONEME:[2]

6.43%; fourth in order of occurrence

VISUAL INTELLIGIBILITY:[3]

12% to 50%; composite 38%

VISUAL CONFUSION:[4]

/t, d, n, l/ (*t*o, *d*o, *n*o, *l*et)

AUDITORY INTELLIGIBILITY IN MILD-TO-SEVERE HEARING IMPAIRMENTS:[5]

79%

AUDITORY CONFUSION:[6]

/m, n, ŋ/ (*m*e, *n*o, si*ng*)

RELATIVE PHONETIC POWER:[7]

36 (range of 1 to 680)

PHONEMIC CONFUSION:[8]

/n/ (*n*o); /ŋ/ (si*ng*); /d/ (*d*o); /dʒ/ (*j*am)

TYPICAL SPELLING:

gn (*gn*aw); *gne* (colo*gne*); *kn* (*kn*ife); *mn* (*mn*emonic); *mp* (co*mp*troller); *n* (*n*o); *ne* (ni*ne*); *nn* (i*nn*); *nne* (A*nne*); *pn* (*pn*eumonia)

/n/ (*no*) PRACTICE MATERIALS

The sound to be stimulated is /n/ (*n*o). Only those words and phrases in which the respondent can articulate all of the sounds correctly, except for the target phoneme, should be utilized for practice. The same stipulation applies to the practice materials provided at the end of this Section.

/ɑ/ knot, nod, nob, wan; /u/ noon, new, Knut, nude; /i/ neat, bean, peanut, seen; /ɑu/ now, down, town, frown; /ɑi/ night, nine, ninth, dine; /ju/ useful, union, unify; /ou/ no, own, known, moan; /ei/ name, pain, rain, feign; /ɔ/ gnaw, dawn, want, awning; /ɔi/ noise, coin, annoy, join; /ɪ/ nip, win, tin, bin; /ɛ/ Nell, Ned, pen, many; /æ/ nap, tan, Dan, hand; /ʊ/ nook; /ʌ/ nut, nothing, ton, Monday; /ə/ minute, another, annoy, China; /ɝ/ burn, turn, journal, colonel; /ɚ/ spinner, mannerly, govern, southern. *Phrases:* The colonel went to

---

1-8 *Ibid.* (see p. 79).

China. It won't be needed for another minute. The wind at dawn is nippy.

Stimulation Unit 19

Phonetic Symbol and Representative Word: /ŋ/ (si*ng*)

Symbol Systems

International Phonetic Alphabet: /ŋ/
Webster's New Collegiate Dictionary (1965): ŋ
Thorndike-Barnhardt Comprehensive Dictionary (1951): ng
Northampton Charts (Yale, 1946): ng

Topographical Relationships of Phoneme Production
/ŋ/ (si*ng*) voiced lingua-velar nasal continuant

MANDIBLE:
slightly lowered
LIPS:
neutral position
TONGUE:
Tip—lowered to position at base of lower front teeth
Back—raised to press against velum or soft palate
AIRSTREAM:
emitted through nasal passages
NASAL PORT:
open
VOCAL FOLDS:
vibrating

Stimulation Procedures

VISUAL-AUDITORY MODEL. A model demonstration is provided by the manipulation of the stimulator's face while the respondent observes. An auditory stimulus is usually given simultaneously as the stimulator is saying: "We are going to say /ŋ/ (si*ng*)." This step may be repeated.

STARTING POSITION. Respondent's articulators should be in the starting position before the manipulation is initiated: lips parted, mandible lowered slightly from position of closure, tongue in customary, relaxed position, vocal folds not vibrating.

SIMULTANEOUS STIMULATION. Stimulator places fingers in position on respondent's face. As the manipulation takes place, the respondent may observe the stimulator's face and/or hear an auditory stimulus.

EXTRAORAL MANIPULATION /ŋ/ (si*ng*)

1. Assume starting position.
2. Extend chin slightly.
3. Gently place finger of one hand on side of nose as a signal for nasal emission of air.
4. Place thumb and middle finger on submandibular points 3 (or use third and ring fingers with palm upward to provide scissors movement).
5. Firmly but gently press upward and inward.
6. Phonate.

If the respondent is in a reclining position, it sometimes facilitates the stimulation of the /ŋ/ (si*ng*).

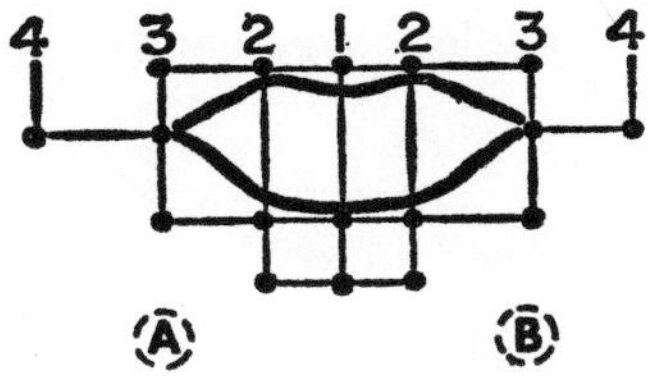

MANIPULATION MODEL: LIPS FORMAT.

/ŋ/ (si*ng*) Response Analysis and Extraoral Cues

TONGUE. /ŋ/ (si*ng*) will be pronounced /ŋg/, if the back of the tongue is lowered while the vocal folds are vibrating. Thus, singing becomes /sɪŋgɪŋg/. If the back of the tongue is lowered suddenly with a slight explosive quality, a voiceless /k/ will be added, thus saying /θɪŋk/ for *thing*.

Often the /n/ (*n*o) will be substituted for /ŋ/ (si*ng*) making humming become /hʌmɪn/ if the tip of the tongue moves upward to /n/ (*n*o) position instead of placing the back of the tongue against the soft palate.

NASAL PORT. If the nasal port is closed during articulation, a /g/ (*g*o) will be substituted.

Closure or obstruction of the vocal port can result in a denasalized quality.

Touching the respondent's larynx with a finger can serve as a signal for phonation.

/ŋ/ (si*ng*) PHONODENTAL GUIDES

Chapter 5 gives details concerning preparation and placement of phonodental guides. Figures 5 and 7 in Chapter 5 illustrate the approximate points of lingual contact for the guides.

Phonodental guides and intraoral cues may be used independently or in combination with the extraoral manipulations. If intraoral stimulation is needed, one or more of the following phonodental guides may be utilized.

Dental Floss Guides /ŋ/ (si*ng*)

Raise tongue sides: two knotted dental floss guides placed between Maxillary First Molars and Second Molars (16-17 and 26-27) or a stretched dental floss guide across Maxillary Second Molars (17 and 27). These guides are difficult to place so deep within the oral cavity. Use of the single long-stemmed wire guide or cue sticks is suggested.

Stemmed Wire Guides /ŋ/ (si*ng*)

Raise back of tongue: single long-stemmed wire guide touches area of lingua-velar contact.

Cue Sticks /ŋ/ (si*ng*)

Cotton-tipped sticks dipped in cold water or parts of tongue depressors may be used to stimulate the same points for lingual contact as those given above.

/ŋ/ (si*ng*) SELECTED PHONEME CHARACTERISTICS

DEVELOPMENTAL AGE:[1]

-ng-, -ng, -ngk = 3 yrs.; -ngkl, -nggl = 6 yrs.

FREQUENCY OF OCCURRENCE OF PHONEME:[2]

1.27% thirty-second in order of occurrence

VISUAL INTELLIGIBILITY:[3]

not given

VISUAL CONFUSION:[4]

not given

AUDITORY INTELLIGIBILITY IN MILD-TO-SEVERE HEARING IMPAIRMENTS:[5]

72%

AUDITORY CONFUSION:[6]

/m, n, ŋ/ (*m*e, *n*o, si*ng*)

RELATIVE PHONETIC POWER:[7]

73 (range of 1 to 680)

PHONEMIC CONFUSION:[8]

/ŋ/ (si*ng*); /n/ (*n*o); /g/ (*g*o)

TYPICAL SPELLING:

n (thi*n*k); *ng* (thi*ng*); *ngue* (to*ngue*)

[1-8] *Ibid.* (see p. 79).

/ŋ/ (*sing*) PRACTICE MATERIALS

The sound to be stimulated is /ŋ/ (*sing*). Only those words and phrases in which the respondent can articulate all of the sounds correctly, except for the target phoneme, should be utilized or practiced. The same stipulation applies to the practice materials provided at the end of this Section.

/ŋ/ (*sing*); /ɑ/ Hong Kong, song, donkey, ping pong; /ɪ/ ping, winging, sing, thing, singer; /æ/ bang, sang, tang, hanger, bank; /ʌ/ Young, tongue, sung, lungs, bunk, youngest; /ɚ/ singer, hanger; *Phrases:* They play ping pong in Hong Kong. The youngest singer lay in the bunk. Bang on the side of the hanger.

COMPARATIVE PRACTICE MATERIALS

Section E: Nasal Continuants

The sounds to be stimulated are /m, n, ŋ/ (*me*, *no*, *sing*). Only those words and phrases in which the respondent can articulate all of the sounds correctly, except for the target phoneme, should be utilized for practice.

	/m/ (*me*)	/n/ (*no*)	/ŋ/ (*sing*)
Initial Position:	me	knee	
	my	nigh	
	may	neigh	
	more	nor	
	mine	nine	
Medial Position:		sinning	singing
		pinning	pinging
		winning	winging
Final Position:	mime	mine	
	tam	tan	Tang
	Sam		sang
	ram	ran	rang

SECTION F: STOP PLOSIVES

Representative Words:	*p*at	*b*e	*t*o	*d*o	*k*eep	*g*o
International Phonetic Alphabet:	p	b	t	d	k	g
Webster's New Collegiate Dictionary (1965):	p	b	t	d	k	g

Thorndike-Barnhardt Comprehensive Dictionary (1951):	p	b	t	d	k	g
Northampton Charts (Yale 1946):	p	d	t	d	k	g

The stop is a sound formed by the complete stoppage of the breath stream at the point of articulation and at the larynx. The air is stopped then suddenly released. The voiced and voiceless pairs of stops (interchangeably called plosives and explosives), /p-b, t-d, k-g/ (*p*at-*b*e, *t*o-*d*o, *k*eep-go) have many characteristics in common:

1. The airstream must be completely stopped.
2. The sound must be suddenly released.
3. The treatment of the aspirate or breathy quality is the same for each pair.
4. One of each pair is voiced.

In understanding the plosive sounds, it is necessary to understand the principle of aspiration. In the three homorganic pairs /p-b, t-d, k-g/, the aspirate or breathy quality, and the vibration or lack of vibration, of the vocal folds are important in distinguishing meaning. Aspiration is the slight puff of breath that immediately follows the explosion. It is an important factor in distinguishing between such words as *bin* and *pin, Tim* and *dim, Kay* and *gay.*

The voiceless plosives /p-t-k/ have more aspiration than their voiced counterparts and are said with a noticeable amount of aspiration /p^h, t^h, k^h/. *For practice stimulation,* however, it is necessary to follow the three steps of forming an explosive sound—namely, directing the airstream toward the point of proper articulators, impounding the air, then exploding it.

The /p/ (*p*at), /b/ (*b*e), /t/ (*t*o), /d/ (*d*o), /k/ (*k*eep), and /g/ (go) are among the most frequently used sounds in English. All these plosives are found in the initial, medial, and final positions of words. The Stimulation Units go from the more visible sounds /p-b/, to the less visible /t-d/, to the back pair /k-g/, that are even less visible.

Stimulation Unit 20

Phonetic Symbol and Representative Word: /p, b/ (*p*at, *b*e)

Symbol Systems

International Phonetic Alphabet: /p, b/
Webster's New Collegiate Dictionary (1965): p, b
Thorndike-Barnhardt Comprehensive Dictionary (1951): p, b
Northampton Charts (Yale, 1946): p, b

Topographical Relationships of Phoneme Production
/p/ (*p*at) voiceless bilabial stop plosive
/b/ (*b*e) voiced bilabial stop plosive

MANDIBLE:
slightly lowered
LIPS:
closed—air compressed at lips, then suddenly released
TONGUE:
neutral position
AIRSTREAM:
emitted through mouth
NASAL PORT:
closed
VOCAL FOLDS:
/p/(*p*at) not vibrating; /b/ (*b*e) vibrating

Stimulation Procedures

VISUAL-AUDITORY MODEL. A model demonstration is provided by the manipulation of the stimulator's face while the respondent observes. An auditory stimulus is usually given simultaneously as the stimulator is saying: "We are going to say /p/ (*p*at) or /b/ (*b*e)." This step may be repeated.

STARTING POSITION. Respondent's articulators should be in the starting position before the manipulation is initiated: lips parted, mandible lowered slightly from position of closure, tongue in customary, relaxed position, vocal folds not vibrating.

SIMULTANEOUS STIMULATION. Stimulator places fingers in position on respondent's face. As the manipulation takes place, the respondent may observe the stimulator's face and/or hear an auditory stimulus.

EXTRAORAL MANIPULATION /p/ (*p*at)

1. Assume starting position.
2. Place thumb and middle finger of one hand on lower lip points 2.
3. Bring lower lip up until it presses on the upper lip.
4. When there is sufficient pressure, fingers on the lower lip bring the mandible downward suddenly into the position for the following sound.
5. An explosion occurs.

If the above manipulation is not sufficient, use the additional manipulation procedures.

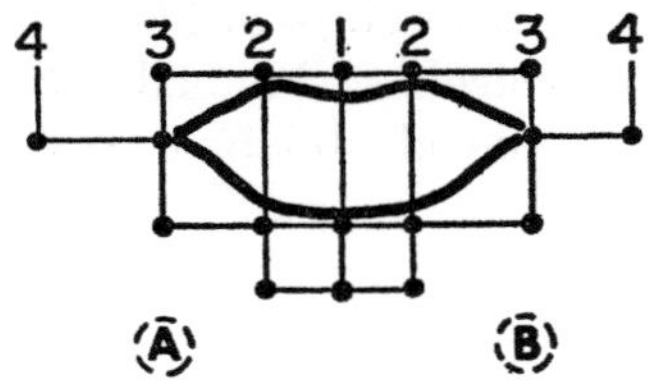

MANIPULATION MODEL: LIPS FORMAT.

ADDITIONAL MANIPULATION

1. Return to starting position.
2. Place the hand not manipulating the lower lip above the respondent's waistline and move it inward with a quick, gentle movement just as the first hand brings the mandible downward, thus facilitating a puff of air.
3. The /ɑ/ (c*a*lm, l*o*t) sound may be combined with the /p/ (*p*at). It is desirable to produce a syllable rather than a single sound, except in cases of such severe impairment that the respondent must concentrate upon a single sound /p/ or /pə/ before attempting a syllable /pɑ/.
4. Add the /ɑ/ (c*a*lm, l*o*t) sound which often facilitates the plosive quality of the /p/ (*p*at) sound because of the extreme position of the mandible when producing the /ɑ/ (c*a*lm, l*o*t).

EXTRAORAL MANIPULATION /b/ (*b*e)

1. Assume starting position.
2. Place thumb and middle finger of one hand on lower lip points 2.
3. Place thumb and middle finger of other hand on upper lip points 2.
4. Press lower and upper lips together and with slightly greater duration as well as with sufficient pressure to produce a plosion upon separation.
5. Phonation begins.
6. Build pressure behind lips.
7. Remove fingers of upper hand.
8. Fingers of lower hand direct the mandible downward suddenly, into position for the following sound.

If the above manipulation is not sufficient, use the additional manipulation procedures.

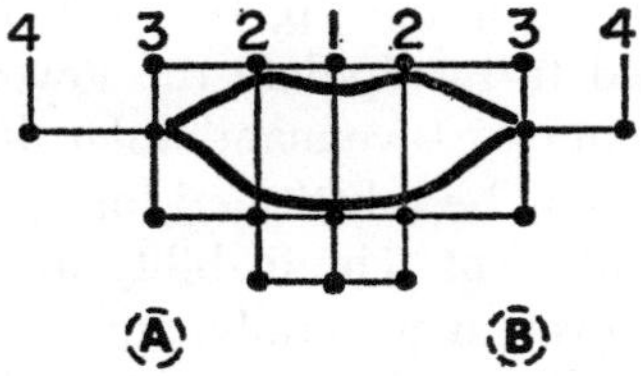

MANIPULATION MODEL: LIPS FORMAT.

ADDITIONAL MANIPULATION

1. Return to starting position.
2. When the /b/ (*b*e) is in final position of a word, do not move the lower lip downward. The lips should be allowed to part without further sound after the beginning of the /b/ (*b*e) is heard. This avoids the additional sound that often accompanies the /b/ (*b*e) sound in the speech of deaf persons.
3. In stimulating the /p/ (*p*at) sound, the lower lip is raised against the upper lip; in the /b/ (*b*e) sound, the lips should be pressed together with equal firmness and for the normal duration of the sound.
4. After the respondent is able to produce the /b/ (*b*e) reasonably well, it is possible to use the sides of the index finger and the thumb of one hand to press the lips together.
5. In the initial position, the /b/ (*b*e) may be combined with /ɑ/ (c*a*lm, l*o*t) in order to feel the forceful separation. The extreme position of /ɑ/ (c*a*lm, l*o*t) seems to facilitate the achievement of the plosive quality of the /b/ (*b*e).
6. The manipulation position for the /b/ (*b*e) is held until vibrations of voicing and backed-up air are felt and then released without pulling the lips apart as in /p/ (*p*at). The voiced /b/ (*b*e) requires a slightly longer holding time than the voiceless /p/ (*p*at) sound.
7. If respondent is able to move the lips rapidly, a series of /p/ (*p*at) and /b/ (*b*e) sounds may be practiced. Add /ɑ/ (c*a*lm, l*o*t) to /p/ (*p*at) and /b/ (*b*e) to produce an easy syllable for initial practice of the manipulation procedures. A schwa sound /ə/ (sof*a*) may be heard with a rapid series of /p/ (*p*at) or /b/ (*b*e).

/p, b/ (*p*at, *b*e) Response Analysis and Extraoral Cues

MANDIBLE. If there is a tendency for the mandible to be lowered more than is appropriate for the /p, b/ (*p*at, *b*e) sounds, the little finger of the hand used to manipulate the lower lip may be hooked under the chin to prevent excessive mandibular depression.

Lips. The /h/ (hat) may be substituted for /p/ (*p*at) or /b/ (*b*at), if the lip contact is insufficient. The inability to produce a satisfactory /p, b/ (*p*at, *b*e), however, is generally caused by incompleteness of the obstruction of the air or the failure to release the sound with enough vigor to produce a plosive quality. A weak emission may give the impression of an omission. The upper lip should not be pulled down for the production of /p/ (*p*at) or /b/ (*b*e).

The finger of the respondent may be placed between the lips of the stimulator to detect the various degrees of pressure and to identify the one that is appropriate for the /p/ (*p*at), /b/ (*b*e), and /m/ (*m*e).

If the lip pressure is too great, it may cause a /p/ (*p*at) or /b/ (*b*e) to be added after the /m/ (*m*e) as in /mbi/ for *me*.

Tongue. There is no contact of the tongue with the upper molars.

Cheeks. The cheeks should not be puffed out in the production of /m, p, b/ (*m*e, *p*at, *b*e). Pressing a thumb and finger against the cheeks can reduce puffing.

Nasal Port. The nostrils may be closed if there is difficulty in producing the /p/ (*p*at) sound.

A mirror may be placed beneath the nostrils of the respondent or stimulator to illustrate the moisture caused by the nasal emission of the /m/ (*m*e) in contrast with the /p/ (*p*at) and /b/ (*b*e).

Airstream. The air pressure needed for /b/ (*b*e) is somewhat less than for /p/ (*p*at). Since /b/ (*b*e) is a voiced sound, little aspiration is expected. A finger of the respondent may be placed against his nose and that of the stimulator to feel the resonance change when /m/ (*m*e) is alternated with /p/ (*p*at) and /b/ (*b*e). The important factor in the pronunciation of /p/ (*p*at) and /b/ (*b*e) is the impounding of air and sudden releases of the impounded air plus vibration of vocal folds on /b/ (*b*e).

A feather or small strip of paper may be held in front of the lips of the respondent or stimulator to compare the degree of explosiveness of /p/ (*p*at) and /b/ (*b*e), or lack of it, on /m/ (*m*e).

Vocal Folds. Continued voicing of the /b/ (*b*e) after the articulators assume a different position will cause a vowel or other sound to be added to the /m/ (*m*e). This problem is common in the speech of many deaf persons.

A finger may be placed on the respondent's larynx to signal phonation for /b/ (*b*e).

/p, b/ (*p*at, *b*e) SELECTED PHONEME CHARACTERISTICS

DEVELOPMENTAL AGE:[1]

p-, -p-, -p = 3 yrs.; -mp, -pt, -pr = 3.5 yrs.; pl-, pr-, sp-, -lp, -mpts, -mps = 4 yrs.; -rp = 5 yrs.; -pl = 6 yrs.; spl-, spr- = 7 yrs.; -sp = 8 yrs.

b-, -b- = 3 yrs.; -br = 3.5 yrs.; -b, bl-, br- = 4 yrs.; -lb, -mbr = 5 yrs.; -rb, -bl = 6 yrs. (not reported: -bd, -rbd.)

FREQUENCY OF OCCURRENCE OF PHONEME:[2]

/p/ 1.37%; thirtieth in order of occurrence
/b/ 1.44%; twenty-eighth in order of occurrence

VISUAL INTELLIGIBILITY:[3]

/p/ 32% to 100%; composite 69%
/b/ 27% to 100%; composite 67%

VISUAL CONFUSION:[4]

/p, b, m/ (*p*at, *b*e, *m*e); /p, w, hw/ (*p*at, *w*e, *wh*at)

AUDITORY INTELLIGIBILITY IN MILD-TO-SEVERE HEARING IMPAIRMENTS:[5]

/p/ 83%
/b/ 66%

AUDITORY CONFUSION:[6]

/p, t, k, h/ (*p*at, *t*o, *k*eep, *h*at);
/b, d, g/ (*b*e, *d*o, *g*o)

RELATIVE PHONETIC POWER:[7]

/p/ 6: /b/ 7 (range of 1 to 680)

PHONEMIC CONFUSION:[8]

/p/ (*p*at); /f/ (*f*ace); /b/ (*b*e), /m/ (*m*e), /v/ (*v*an)

TYPICAL SPELLING:

/p/ *p* (*p*ie), *pe* (ca*pe*), *pp* (ha*pp*y), *gh* (hiccou*gh*), *ph* (she*ph*erd); /b/ *b* (*b*a*b*y), *bb* (e*bb*), *be* (ro*be*)

/p, b/ (*p*at, *b*e) PRACTICE MATERIALS

The sounds to be stimulated are /p/ (*p*at) and /b/ (*b*e). Only those words and phrases in which the respondent can articulate all of the sounds correctly, except the target phoneme, should be utilized for practice. The same stipulation applies to the practice materials provided at the end of this Section.

/p/ (*p*at)

/ɑ/ palm, pot, hop, upon; /u/ pool, loop, soup, approve; /i/ peak,

[1-8] *Ibid.* (see p. 79).

peach, keep, peace; /ɑu/ power, pouch, Powell, impound; /ɑi/ pine, pie, ripe, Magpie; /iu/ puma, dupe, dispute; /ou/ pony, pole, rope, suppose; /ei/ paper, pay, tape, repay; /ɔ/ Paul, paw, pauper, pawpaw; /ɔi/ poi, appoint; /ɪ/ pin, pig, ship, hippy; /ɛ/ pet, pep, peppy, carpet; /æ/ pan, pal, rap, repast; /ʊ/ pull, put, push, pulpit; /ʌ/ puff, pup, up, guppy; /ɝ/ purr, person, purple, perch; /ɚ/ paper, keeper, supper, deeper. *Phrases:* Pam types. Pam helped pack the carpets. Soup and pumpkin pie appeal to Paul.

/b/ (*b*e)

/ɑ/ bomb, Bobby, cob, anybody; /u/ boom, booth, tube; /i/ beat, be, because, bean; /ɑu/ bough, Baum, bower, about; /ɑi/ buy, bite, jibe, bye-bye; /iu/ Beulah, tube, cube; /ou/ boat, both, robe, about; /ei/ bate, bay, Abe, baby; /ɔ/ ball, football; /ɔi/ boy, boil, highboy, doughboy; /ɪ/ bill, beer, rib, rabbit; /ɛ/ bare, bed, web, Debbie; /æ/ bad, bag, cab, gabby; /ʊ/ book, bush, bull, boor; /ʌ/ bun, bug, tub, above; /ə/ ribbon, gibbon, cherub, Sheba; /ɝ/ bird, burr, curb, rebirth; /ɚ/ number, robber, labor, liberty. *Phrases:* Ben's big brother bought the boat. Bob batted the baseball. Nobody remembers Babs.

Stimulation Unit 21

Phonetic Symbol and Representative Word: /t, d/ (*t*o, *d*o)

Symbol Systems

International Phonetic Alphabet: /t, d/
Webster's New Collegiate Dictionary (1965): t, d
Thorndike-Barnhardt Comprehensive Dictionary (1951): t, d
Northampton Charts (Yale, 1946): t, d

Topographical Relationships of Phoneme Production

/t/ (*t*o) voiceless lingua-alveolar stop plosive
/d/ (*d*o) voiced lingua-alveolar stop plosive

MANDIBLE:
slightly lowered

LIPS:
slightly open and everted to follow line of depression of mandible

TONGUE:
Tip—raised to make contact with alveolar ridge back of upper front teeth where air is compressed
Sides—in contact with upper teeth

AIRSTREAM:
emitted through mouth
NASAL PORT:
closed
VOCAL FOLDS:
/t/ not vibrating; /d/ vibrating

Stimulation Procedures

VISUAL-AUDITORY MODEL. A model demonstration is provided by the manipulation of the stimulator's face while the respondent observes. An auditory stimulus is usually given simultaneously as the stimulator is saying: "We are going to say /t/ (*t*o) or /d/ (*d*o)." This step may be repeated

STARTING POSITION. Respondent's articulators should be in the starting position before the manipulation is initiated: lips parted; mandible lowered slightly from position of closure; tongue in customary, relaxed position; vocal folds not vibrating.

SIMULTANEOUS STIMULATION. Stimulator places fingers in position on respondent's face. As the manipulation takes place, the respondent may observe the stimulator's face and/or hear an auditory stimulus.

EXTRAORAL MANIPULATION /t/ (*t*o)

1. Assume starting position.
2. Place index finger of same or of other hand on upper lip point 1.
3. Exert slight pressure.
4. Remove finger with flicking motion.

EXTRAORAL MANIPULATION /d/ (*d*o)

1. Assume starting position.
2. Place second finger of other hand on upper lip point 1.
3. Press firmly and with slightly greater duration.
4. Remove finger with flicking motion as soon as
5. Phonation begins. (The Stimulator may signal phonation by placing little finger against respondent's larynx.)

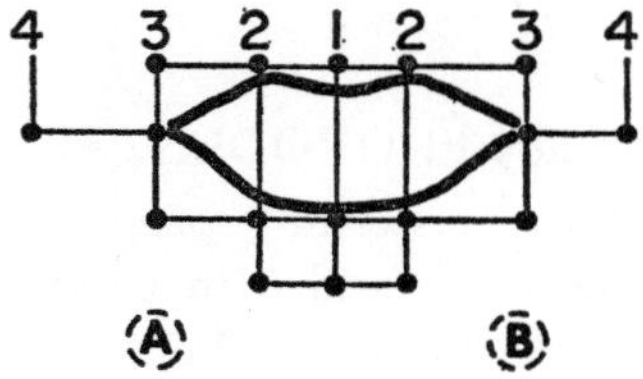

MANIPULATION MODEL: LIPS FORMAT.

/t, d/ (*to*, *do*) Response Analysis and Extraoral Cues

MANDIBLE. The mandible may be dropped inappropriately for the /n, t, d/ (*no*, *to*, *do*) when these sounds are produced with the tongue tip down and the forward part of the tongue body obstructs the air by pressing against the alveolar ridge.

TONGUE. If the tongue tip is protruded or touches the back of the incisors, a thickened sound resembling the /θ/ (*th*in) may result. This position diminishes the plosive quality. This position is unattractive and may complicate the combining of the /n, t, d/ (*no*, *to*, *do*) with following sounds.

The /t/ (*to*) that is produced farther back than the alveolar ridge is called an inverted or retroflex /t/ (*to*). A sound resembling an /s/ (*so*) may result if the tongue tip contact is not complete, there is insufficient pressure, or there is a slow release of the final /t/ (*to*).

When the tip of the tongue is placed behind the lower incisors, the lingual contact with the upper incisors is made with the body of the tongue.

NASAL PORT. Deaf children frequently nasalize /d/ (*do*). They may see the tongue drop for the production of the /t/ (*to*) without realizing the need for sufficient pressure to produce the plosive characteristics of the /t/ (*to*).

AIRSTREAM. A vowel should not be heard after final /t/ (a*t*). The vowel murmur /ə/ may be heard after /d/ (a*dd*), and /n/ (o*n*).

When the /d/ (*do*) is followed by a second plosive sound, only one plosive is heard and one explosion occurs as in *bedding* and *tadpole*. This is true for all plosives.

The fingers of the respondent may be held in front of his open lips and/or those of the stimulator so the contrasting degree of plosiveness can be detected.

VOCAL FOLDS. There is a tendency to voice the /t/ (*to*) when it appears between two voiced sounds. This results in a /d/ (*do*) sound as in *city*. Omission of final /t/ (a*t*) in voiceless consonant blends such as *best, fact, slept,* should be avoided.

A finger may be placed against the respondent's larynx to signal phonation.

/t, d/ (*to*, *do*) PHONODENTAL GUIDES

Chapter 5 gives details concerning preparation and placement of phonodental guides. Figures 5 and 6 in Chapter 5 illustrate the approximate points of lingual contact for the guides.

Phonodental guides and intraoral cues may be used independently or in combination with the extraoral manipulations.

The extraoral manipulation is usually effective for eliciting this phoneme, and intraoral stimulation is not required. If intraoral stimulation is needed, one or more of the following phonodental guides may be utilized.

Denture Guides /t, d/ (*t*o, *d*o)
Raise tongue tip: one guide placed between Maxillary Central Incisors (11-21).

Dental Floss Guides /t, d/ (*t*o, *d*o)
Raise tongue tip: one knotted dental floss guide placed between Maxillary Central Incisors (11-21).

Stemmed Wire Guides /t, d/ (*t*o, *d*o)
Raise tongue tip: longer stem of double-ended stemmed wire guide used to position tongue tip behind Maxillary Central Incisors (11-21).

Cue Sticks /t, d/ (*t*o, *d*o)
Cotton-tipped sticks dipped in cold water or parts of tongue depressors may be used to stimulate the same points for lingual contact as those given above.

/t, d/ (*t*o, *d*o) SELECTED PHONEME CHARACTERISTICS

DEVELOPMENTAL AGE:[1]

/t/ t-, -t = 3 yrs.; -pt = 3.5 yrs.; tr-, tw-, st-, -rt, -ft, -lt, -mpt = 4 yrs.; str- = 5 yrs.; -t-, -nt, -str, -rst, -ntth, = 6 yrs.; -st, -kst, = 7 yrs.; -kt, -tr = 8 yrs.; -tl not produced correctly by 75% of children by 8 years of age.

/d/ d-, -d-, = 3 yrs.; -dr = 3.5 yrs.; -d, dr- = 4 yrs.; -rd = 5 yrs.; -nd = 6 yrs.

FREQUENCY OF OCCURRENCE OF PHONEME:[2]

/t/ 9.11%; second in order of occurrence
/d/ 3.78%; fifth in order of occurrence

VISUAL INTELLIGIBILITY:[3]

/t/ 26% to 56%; composite 42%
/d/ 9% to 50%; composite 36%

VISUAL CONFUSION:[4]

/t, d, n, l/ (*t*o, *d*o, *n*o, *l*et)

AUDITORY INTELLIGIBILITY IN MILD-TO-SEVERE HEARING IMPAIRMENTS:[5]

/t/ 73%
/d/ 69%

AUDITORY CONFUSION:[6]

/b, d, g/ (*b*e, *d*o, *g*o); /p, t, k, h/ (*p*at, *t*o, *k*eep, *h*at)

Relative Phonetic Power:[7]

/t/ 15; /d/ 7 (range of 1 to 680)

Phonemic Confusion:[8]

/t/ (*t*o), /k/ (*k*eep), /θ/ (*th*in), /s/ (*s*o), /tʃ/ (*ch*in), /d/ (*d*o), /g/ (go), /ð/ (*th*is), /z/ (*z*one), /dʒ/ (*j*am)

Typical Spelling:

/t/ *bt* (de*bt*); *cht* (ya*cht*); *ct* (indi*ct*); *ed* (ask*ed*); *ght* (bou*ght*); *phth* (*phth*isic); *pt* (recei*pt*); *t* (*t*all); *te* (ki*te*); *th* (*th*yme); *tt* (ma*tt*er); *tte* (dine*tte*); *tw* (*tw*o); /d/ *d* (*d*o); *dd* (la*dd*er) *de* (ma*de*); *ed* (order*ed*)

/t, d/ (*t*o, *d*o) PRACTICE MATERIALS

The sounds to be stimulated are /t/ (*t*o) and /d/ (*d*o). Only those words and phrases in which the respondent can articulate all of the sounds correctly, except the target phoneme, should be utilized for practice. The same stipulation applies to the practice materials provided at the end of this Section.

/t/ (*t*o)

/ɑ/ Tom, hot, not, tick-tock; /u/ to, boot, root, retool; /i/ team, teeth, meat, beating; /ɑu/ town, tower, about, doubtful; /ɑi/ time, tight, might, untie; /iu/ tune, tube, beautify; /ou/ toe, tone, boat, toad; /ei/ table, ate, gate, tomato; /ɔ/ tall, bought, thought, talks; /ɔi/ toy, toil, Hoyt, loiter; /ɪ/ tin, tick, pit, pretty; /ɛ/ tell, ten, net, Betty; /æ/ tan, gnat, at, attack, /ʊ/ took, tour, put, undertook; /ʌ/ ton, tub, cut, putt; /ə/ today, basket, metal, bottom; /ɝ/ terms, turn, Bert, return; /ɚ/ letter, butter, water, hotter. *Phrases:* Kate's late to the tea. Pete eats meat on Tuesday. It is difficult to tell time.

/d/ (*d*o)

/ɑ/ Don, dog, nod, model; /u/ duke, do, food, voodoo; /i/ dean, deep, need, indeed; /ɑu/ down, dour, loud, rowdy; /ɑi/ die, dime, tied, Heidi; /iu/ duke, due, endure; /ou/ dome, mode, road, dodo; /ei/ day, dame, made, radio; /ɔ/ door, laud, audible; /ɔi/ Boyd, Lloyd, overjoyed; /ɪ/ dim, Dick, did, endear; /ɛ/ den, Ted, said, ready; /æ/ Dan, daddy, sad, candy; /ʊ/ during, could, should, wooden; /ʌ/ Doug, duck, bud, sudden; /ə/ Adam, sudden, garden, widen; /ɝ/ dirt, bird, word, herded; /ɚ/ under, herder, girder. *Phrases:* Andy stood ready at the door. Dan ducked behind the studio door. Dot read out loud.

[1-8] *Ibid.* (see p. 79).

Stimulation Unit 22

Phonetic Symbol and Representative Word: /k, g/ (*k*eep, go)

Symbol Systems

International Phonetic Alphabet: /k, g/
Webster's New Collegiate Dictionary (1965): k, g
Thorndike-Barnhardt Comprehensive Dictionary (1951): k, g
Northampton Charts (Yale, 1946): k, g

Topographical Relationships of Phoneme Production

/k/ (*k*eep)	voiceless	lingua-velar	stop plosive
/g/ (go)	voiced	lingua-velar	stop plosive

MANDIBLE:
slightly lowered

LIPS:
neutral position

TONGUE:
Tip—lowered to position at base of lower front teeth
Back—raised to press against velum or soft palate, thus causing airstream to be momentarily stopped. There is compression of airstream; the back of the tongue is suddenly dropped permitting release of compressed air

AIRSTREAM:
emitted through mouth

NASAL PORT:
closed

VOCAL FOLDS:
/k/ not vibrating; /g/ vibrating

Stimulation Procedures

VISUAL-AUDITORY MODEL. A model demonstration is provided by the manipulation of the stimulator's face while the respondent observes. An auditory stimulus is usually given simultaneously as the stimulator is saying: "We are going to say /k/ (*k*eep) or /g/ (go).

STARTING POSITION. Respondent's articulator's should be in the starting position before the manipulation is initiated: lips parted; mandible lowered slightly from position of closure; tongue in customary, relaxed position; vocal folds not vibrating.

SIMULTANEOUS STIMULATION. Stimulator places fingers in position on respondent's face. As the manipulation takes place, the respondent may observe the stimulator's face and/or hear an auditory stimulus.

EXTRAORAL MANIPULATION /k/ (*k*eep)

1. Assume starting position.
2. Place thumb and middle finger on submandibular points 3 (or use middle and ring fingers with palm upward) in preparation for scissors movement.
3. Press upward and inward firmly but gently.
4. Release as soon as the back of tongue has reached velar contact.

If the above manipulation is not sufficient, use the additional manipulation procedures.

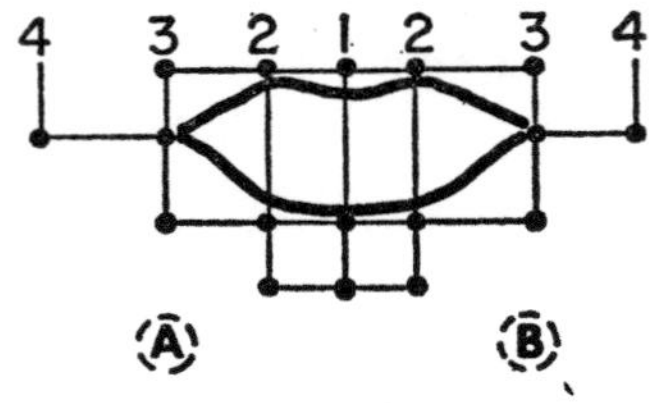

MANIPULATION MODEL: LIPS FORMAT.

ADDITIONAL MANIPULATION

If the /k/ (*k*eep) is to be followed by another sound, use thumb and middle finger of other hand to stimulate second sound. The /ɑ/ (c*a*lm, l*o*t) is usually the easiest to use in initial practice. The exaggerated movement from /k/ (*k*eep) to /ɑ/ (c*a*lm, l*o*t) should facilitate the plosive quality of the /k/ (*k*eep). A schwa may be heard with rapid series of the /k/ (*k*eep) sound.

EXTRAORAL MANIPULATION /g/ (*g*o)

1. Assume starting position.
2. Place thumb and middle finger on submandibular points 3 (or use third and ring fingers with palm upward) in preparation for scissors movement.
3. Press upward and inward firmly and gently.
4. Phonate.
5. Release as soon as the back of tongue has reached velar contact.

If the respondent is in a reclining position, it sometimes facilitates the stimulation of /k, g/ (*k*eep, *g*o).

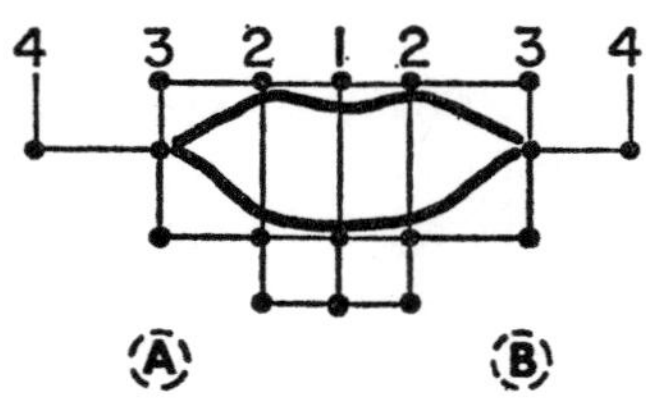

MANIPULATION MODEL: LIPS FORMAT.

/k, g/ (*k*eep, go) Response Analysis and Extraoral Cues

AIRSTREAM. If there is excessive aspiration, it distorts the sound. Excessive aspiration can be used for kinetic reasons during initial practice periods.

Too little aspiration on voiceless /k/ will result in a sound which the English speaker will interpret as /g/, thus *kill* is interpreted as *gill.*

The fingers of the respondent may be held in front of his own open lips and/or those of the stimulator so the contrasting degree of plosiveness can be detected.

VOCAL BANDS. /k/ will become /g/, its voiced counterpart, if vocal folds vibrate. This principle occurs more frequently in a medial position when /k/ comes between two voiced sounds as in *making* /meigɪŋ/.

When /g/ appears in a final position it sometimes becomes unvoiced to /k/ if vocal folds cease to vibrate, thus *beg* /bɛg/ becomes /bɛk/.

Touching the respondent's larynx with a finger can serve as a signal for phonation.

/k, g/ (*k*eep, go) PHONODENTAL GUIDES

Chapter 5 gives details concerning preparation and placement of phonodental guides. Figures 5 and 6 in Chapter 5 illustrate the approximate points of lingual contact for the guides.

Dental Floss Guides /k, g/ (*k*eep, go)

Raise tongue sides: two knotted dental floss guides placed between Maxillary First Molars and Second Molars (16-17 and 26-27); or a stretched dental floss guide across Maxillary Second Molars (17 and 27). These guides are difficult to place so deep within the oral cavity. Use of the long stemmed wire guide or cue stick is suggested.

Stemmed Wire Guides /k, g/ (*k*eep, go)

Raise back of tongue: single long stemmed wire guide touches place of lingua-velar contact.

Cue Sticks /k, g/ (*k*eep, go)

Cotton-tipped sticks dipped in cold water or parts of tongue depressors may be used to stimulate the same points for lingual contact as those given above.

/k, g/ (*k*eep, go) SELECTED PHONEME CHARACTERISTICS

DEVELOPMENTAL AGE:[1]

k-, -k-, ngk = 3 yrs.; -rk, -ks, -kr = 3.5 yrs.; -k, kl-, kr-, kw-, sk- =

4 yrs.; -lk, -kl, skw- ngkl = 6 yrs.; -sk, skr-, -skr, -kst = 7 yrs.; -kt = 8 yrs.

g-, -g- = 3 yrs.; -gr = 3.5 yrs.; -g, gl- = 4 yrs.; gr- = 4.5 yrs.; -rg, -gl, nggl = 6 yrs.

FREQUENCY OF OCCURRENCE OF PHONEME:[2]

/k/ 2.93%; eleventh in order of occurrence

/g/ 1.39%; twenty-ninth in order of occurrence

VISUAL INTELLIGIBILITY:[3]

/k/ 0% to 67%; composite 32%

/g/ 0% to 28%; composite 23%

VISUAL CONFUSION:[4]

/k, g, h/ (*k*eep, go, *h*at)

AUDITORY INTELLIGIBILITY IN MILD-TO-SEVERE HEARING IMPAIRMENTS:[5]

/k/ 63%

/g/ 71%

AUDITORY CONFUSION:[6]

/p, t, k, h/ (*p*at, *t*o, *k*eep, *h*at);

/b, d, g/ (*b*e, *d*o, go)

RELATIVE PHONETIC POWER:[7]

/k/ 13; /g/ 15 (range of 1 to 680)

PHONEMIC CONFUSION:[8]

/k/ (*k*eep), /t/ (*t*o), /ʔ/ (glottal stop); /g/ (go), /d/ (*d*o), /ŋ/ (si*ng*)

TYPICAL SPELLING:

/k/ *c* (*c*at); *cc* (a*cc*ount); *ch* (e*ch*o); *che* (a*che*); *ck* (lu*ck*); *cq* (a*cq*uire); *cque* (sa*cque*); *cu* (bis*cu*it); *k* (*k*it); *ke* (co*ke*); *kh* (*kh*aki); *lk* (fo*lk*); *q* (s*q*uash); *qu* (con*qu*er); *que* (cli*que*); *x* (si*x*ty); /g/ *c* (e*c*zema); *g* (*g*o); *gg* (e*gg*); *gh* (*gh*etto); *gu* (*gu*ide); *gue*(pla*gue*).

/k, g/ (*k*eep, go) PRACTICE MATERIALS

The sounds to be stimulated are /k/ (*k*eep) and /g/ (go). Only those words and phrases in which the respondent can articulate all of the sounds correctly, except the target phoneme, should be utilized for practice. The same stipulation applies to the practice materials provided at the end of this Section.

/k/ (*k*eep)

/ɑ/ calm, con, knock, locker; /u/ coop, cool, duke, lukewarm; /i/ keen, key, cheek, deacon; /ɑu/ cow, couch, cowlick, account; /ɑi/ kine, kite, Mike, hike, unkind; /iu/ cute, cupid, duke, acute; /ou/

[1-8] *Ibid.* (see p. 79).

comb, coat, coke, oak; /ei/ came, cake, overcame, baked; /ɔ/ call, talk, walk, recall; /ɔi/ coin, coy, recoil, decoy; /ɪ/ kit, kiss, chick, kick; /ɛ/ Kelly, care, peck, second; /æ/ can, cat, back, recap; /ʊ/ could, cook, book, cookie; /ʌ/ cup, luck, duck, overcome; /ə/ occur, second, beckon, beacon; /ɝ/ curb, perk, occur, worked. *Phrases:* Nick can't keep a secret. Jack drank coke. Kate called cousin Carl.

/g/ (go)

/ɑ/ got, hog, dog, saga; /u/ goose, goon, Dugan, mongoose; /i/ geese, league, legal, Teague; /ɑu/ gown, gout, nightgown; /ɑi/ guide, guile, guise, bygone; /ou/ goat, goes, vogue, ghost; /ei/ game, gay, gave, regain; /ɔ/ gone, gall, dog, augment; /ɔi/ goiter, Goya; /ɪ/ give, pig, big, buggy; /ɛ/ get, peg, leg, again; /æ/ gap, rag, shag, began; /ʊ/ good, no-good; /ʌ/ gum, gust, bug, airgun; /ə/ organ, legal, pagan, Regan; /ɝ/ gird, girdle, girl, Bergman; /ɚ/ dagger, finger, sugar, beggar. *Phrases:* Gregg's seagulls are hungry. Jay gave Agnes a gift.

COMPARATIVE PRACTICE MATERIALS

SECTION F: STOP PLOSIVE

The sounds to be stimulated are /p, b, t, d, k, g/ (*p*at, *b*e, *t*o, *d*o, *k*eep, *g*o). Only those words and phrases in which the respondent can articulate all of the sounds correctly, except the target phoneme, should be utilized for practice.

	/p/ (*p*at)	/b/ (*b*e)	/t/ (*t*o)	/d/ (*d*o)	/k/ (*k*eep)	/g/ (*g*o)
Initial	pet	bet	Tet	debt	kept	get
Position:	pat	bat	tat	dad	cat	gat
	Poe	bow	toe	doe	Coe	go
	pie	buy	tie	die	kite	guy
	pond	bond		donned	conned	
	peep	beep		deep	keep	
			Etta	Edda	echo	ego
Medial		Abbey		Addie		Aggie
Position:		oboe	oto	Odum	Oakie	
Final	nap	nab	knat	mad	knack	nag
Position:	pup	pub	putt	mud	puck	pug
	cup	cub	cut	cud	luck	lug
	cape	Cabe	Kate	made	cake	egg
	lap	lab	mat	lad	lack	lag

SECTION G: FRICATIVES (PART ONE)

Representative Words:	*h*at	*f*ace	*v*an	*th*in	*th*is
International Phonetic Alphabet:	/h/	/f/	/v/	/θ/	/ð/
Webster's New Collegiate Dictionary (1965):	h	f	v	th	*th*
Thorndike-Barnhardt Comprehensive Dictionary (1951):	h	f	v	th[1]	TH[2]
Northampton Charts (Yale, 1946):	h	f	v	th	th

The glottal, unpaired, voiceless fricative /h/ is the most "backed" of all the English sounds. What we hear for /h/ is a brief glottal friction, instantly abandoned in preparation for producing the following vowel in a word.

The voiced and voiceless pairs of fricatives /f, v/ (*f*ace, *v*an) and /θ, ð/ (*th*in, *th*e), following the articulatory pattern of going from the more fronted labiodental /f, v/ to the linguadental /θ, ð/. These fricatives are "visible" thus adding greater ease of stimulation.

All five of these fricatives are continuants. They are called fricatives because of the friction caused by forcing the breath stream through a small opening between the articulators.

Stimulation Unit 23

Phonetic Symbol and Representative Word: /h/ (*h*at)

Symbol Systems

International Phonetic Alphabet: /h/
Webster's New Collegiate Dictionary (1965): h
Thorndike-Barnhardt Comprehensive Dictionary (1951): h
Northampton Charts (Yale, 1946): h

Topographical Relationships of Phoneme Production
/h/ (*h*at) voiceless glottal fricative continuant

MANDIBLE:
slightly lowered
LIPS:
neutral position

Tongue:
relaxed and neutral
Airstream:
emitted through mouth
Nasal Port:
closed
Vocal Folds:
not vibrating

Stimulation Procedures

Visual-Auditory Model. A model demonstration is provided by the manipulation of the stimulator's face while the respondent observes. An auditory stimulus is usually given simultaneously as the stimulator is saying: "We are going to say /h/ (*h*at)." This step may be repeated.

Starting Position. Respondent's articulators should be in the starting position before the manipulation is initiated: lips parted, mandible lowered slightly from position of closure, tongue in customary, relaxed position, vocal folds not vibrating.

Simultaneous Stimulation. Stimulator places fingers in position on respondent's face. As the manipulation takes place, the respondent may observe the stimulator's face and/or hear an auditory stimulus.

EXTRAORAL MANIPULATION /h/ (*h*at)

1. Assume starting position.
2. Use one hand on chin to lower mandible sufficiently to allow the breath to pass freely through the oral cavity.
3. Use the other hand to press inward and upward with a sudden movement just below the sternum, forcing the diaphram upward.

If the above manipulation is not sufficient, use the additional manipulation procedures.

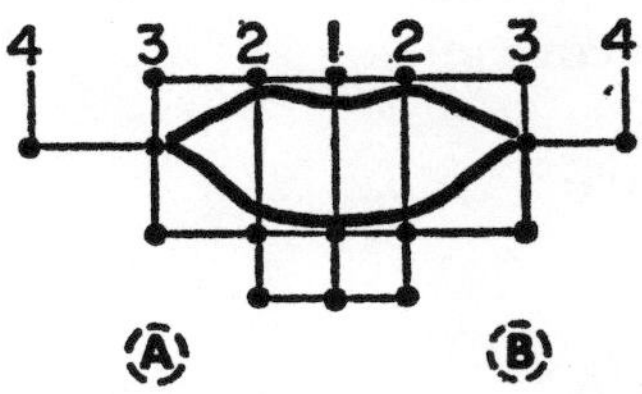

MANIPULATION MODEL: LIPS FORMAT.

ADDITIONAL MANIPULATION

The /h/ (*h*at) is usually followed by a vowel or diphthong, thus a quick adjustment of the mandible to the degree of opening appropriate for the following sound is necessary.

Panting often helps stimulate the /h/ (*h*at).

/h/ (*h*at) Response Analysis and Extraoral Cues

AIRSTREAM. In exerting pressure just below the sternum to force the air out, the stimulator should take care not to apply so much force that it is painful or disagreeable for the respondent.

A strip of paper or feather may be used to demonstrate amount of air flow.

The stimulator may place one hand on the respondent's back so the latter will not recoil or bend forward. It is sometimes easier to stimulate the sound if the respondent is either standing or lying down.

VOCAL FOLDS. Often the respondent adds voicing to the airstream. If this is done, the stimulator should increase the suddenness of the stimulation and add the /ɑ/ (c*a*lm) so that *ha, ha, ha,* is produced. Other vowels may also be used.

/h/ (*h*at) SELECTED PHONEME CHARACTERISTICS

DEVELOPMENTAL AGE:[1]
h-, -h- = 3 years

FREQUENCY OF OCCURRENCE OF PHONEME:[2]
1.49%; twenty-sixth in order of occurrence

VISUAL INTELLIGIBILITY:[3]
0% to 53%; composite 33%

VISUAL CONFUSION:[4]
/k, g, h/ (*k*eep, *g*o, *h*at)

AUDITORY INTELLIGIBILITY IN MILD-TO-SEVERE HEARING IMPAIRMENTS:[5]
58%

AUDITORY CONFUSION:[6]
/p, t, k, h/ (*p*at, *t*o, *k*eep, *h*at)

RELATIVE PHONETIC POWER:[7]
not given

PHONEMIC CONFUSION:[8]
not given

TYPICAL SPELLING:
h (*h*at); *wh* (*wh*o)

[1-8] *Ibid.* (see p. 79).

/h/ (*h*at) PRACTICE MATERIALS

The sound to be stimulated is /h/ (*h*at). Only those words and phrases in which the respondent can articulate all of the sounds, except the target phoneme, should be utilized for practice. The same stipulation applies to the practice materials provided at the end of this Section.

The vowels and diphthongs for use with the target phoneme are arranged so that the most easily stimulated are listed first. This arrangement is compatible with the recommendations given in Chapter 6.

/ɑ/ hop, hot, aha; /u/ who, whom; /i/ heat, heap; /ɑu/ how, howl; /ɑi/ high, height; /iu/ Hugh, hewed; /ou/ hoe, hole, ho-ho; /ei/ hay, hate; /ɔ/ haw, heehaw; /ɔi/ ahoy, Hoyle; /ɪ/ hit, him, adhere; /ɛ/ hem, hen; /æ/ hat, happen; /ʊ/ hook, hood; /ʌ/ hut, hum, /ə/ ahem, ahead; /ɝ/ hurst, herd. *Phrases:* Hugh held the hunting hounds. Helen hemmed the housecoat. He held the hat.

Stimulation Unit 24

Phonetic Symbol and Representative Word: /f, v/ (*f*ace, *v*an)

Symbol Systems

International Phonetic Alphabet: /f, v/
Webster's New Collegiate Dictionary (1965): f, v
Thorndike-Barnhardt Comprehensive Dictionary (1951): f, v
Northampton Charts (Yale, 1946): f, v

Topographical Relationships of Phoneme Production

/f/ (*f*ace) voiceless labio-dental fricative continuant
/v/ (*v*an) voiced labio-dental fricative continuant

MANDIBLE:
raised position to accommodate lower lip

LIPS:
Lower—in contact with edge of upper incisors

TEETH:
Upper—upper incisors in contact with lower lip

TONGUE:
neutral position

AIRSTREAM:
forced through small aperture between teeth and lip

NASAL PORT:
closed

VOCAL FOLDS:
/f/ not vibrating; /v/ vibrating

Stimulation Procedures

VISUAL-AUDITORY MODEL. A model demonstration is provided by the manipulation of the stimulator's face while the respondent observes. An auditory stimulus is usually given simultaneously as the stimulator is saying: "We are going to say /f/ (*f*ace) or /v/ (*v*an)." This step may be repeated.

STARTING POSITION. Respondent's articulators should be in the starting position before the manipulation is initiated: lips parted, mandible lowered slightly from position of closure, tongue in customary, relaxed position, vocal folds not vibrating.

SIMULTANEOUS STIMULATION. Stimulator places fingers in position on respondent's face. As the manipulation takes place, the respondent may observe the stimulator's face and/or hear an auditory stimulus.

EXTRAORAL MANIPULATION /f/ (*f*ace)

1. Assume starting position.
2. Place thumb and middle finger on lower lip line point 2.
3. Move lower lip upward into approximation with edge of upper incisors.
4. Emit airstream through labiodental aperture.
5. Exert slight pressure before removing fingers.

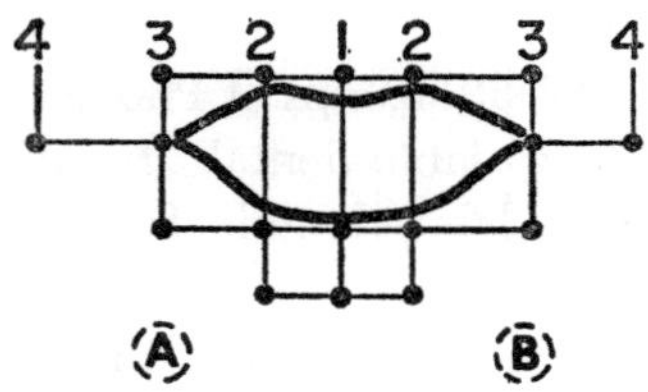

MANIPULATION MODEL: LIPS FORMAT.

EXTRAORAL MANIPULATION /v/ (*v*an)

1. Assume starting position.
2. Place thumb and middle finger on lower lip line points 2.
3. Move lower lip upward into approximation with edge of upper incisors.
4. Emit airstream through labiodental aperture.
5. Press firmly and with slightly greater duration than for the /f/ (*f*ace).
6. Phonate.

If the above manipulations are not sufficient, use the additional procedures.

ADDITIONAL MANIPULATION

1. Return to starting position.
2. Place thumb and middle finger on lower lip line points 2.
3. Place thumb and middle finger of other hand on upper lip line points 2.
4. Raise upper lip sufficiently to avoid contact with lower lip.
5. Move lower lip upward into approximation with edge of upper incisors.
6. Direct the airstream through labiodental aperture.
7. Phonate. (For the /v/ (*v*an) the stimulator may touch the respondent's larynx with the little finger of the lower hand to signal phonation.

Stimulating the /ɑ/ (c*a*lm, l*o*t) after the /f, v/ (*f*ace, *v*an) provides downward manipulation in a direct line.

/f, v/ (*f*ace, *v*an) Response Analysis and Extraoral Cues

Airstream. If initiation of airstream is a problem, use one hand to press gently but firmly at a point just below sternum. This pressure should generate a steady flow of air.

A strip of paper or a feather may be used to demonstrate the desired amount of airflow.

Lips. When the upper lip drops, the labiodental sounds tend to become bilabial.

Vocal Folds. A finger may be placed on the respondent's larynx to signal phonation.

/f, v/ (*f*ace, *v*an) SELECTED PHONEME CHARACTERISTICS

Developmental Age:[1]

f-, -f-, -f = 3 yrs.; -ft, -fr = 4 yrs.; fr-, -lf = 4.5 yrs.; fl-, -rf = 5 yrs.; -fl = 6 yrs.; -v- = 4 yrs.; v-, -v = 6 yrs.

Frequency of Occurrence of Phoneme:[2]

/f/ 83% to 100%; composite 87%

/v/ 1.76%; twenty-fourth in order of occurrence

Visual Intelligibility:[3]

/f/ 83% to 100% composite 87%

/v/ 61% to 100%; composite 72%

Visual Confusion:[4]

/f, v/ (*f*ace, *v*an)

Auditory Intelligibility in Mild-to-Severe Hearing Impairments:[5]

59%; 59%

AUDITORY CONFUSION:[6]

/ʃ, s, f, θ, tʃ/ (*sh*oe, *s*o, *f*ace, *th*in, *ch*in)

/ʒ, z, v, ð, dʒ, j/ (a*z*ure, *z*one, *v*an, *th*is, *j*am, *y*et)

RELATIVE PHONETIC POWER:[7]

/f/ 5; /v/ 12 (range of 1 to 680)

PHONEMIC CONFUSION:[8]

/f/ (face), /p/ (pat), /θ/ (thin), /v/ (van), /b/ (be), /ð/ (*th*is)

TYPICAL SPELLING:

/f/ *f* (*f*ame); *fe* (wi*fe*); *ff* (co*ff*ee); *gh* (lau*gh*); *lf* (ca*lf*); *ph* (*ph*onetic); /v/ *f* (o*f*); *lve* (ha*lve*); *ph* (Ste*ph*en); *v* (*v*ery); *ve* (li*ve*); *vv* (fli*vv*er)

/f, v/ (*f*ace, *v*an) PRACTICE MATERIALS

The sounds to be stimulated are /f/ (*f*ace) and /v/ (*v*an). Only those words and phrases in which the respondent can articulate all of the sounds correctly, except the target phoneme, should be utilized for practice. The same stipulation applies to the practice materials provided at the end of this Section.

/f/ (*f*ace)

/ɑ/ fodder, fond, calf, doff; /u/ food, fool, buffoon, goof; /i/ feel, feed, feet, defeat; /ɑu/ fowl, found, unfounded; /ɑi/ fight, file, defy, fife; /iu/ few, fuel, refuel, refuse; /ou/ foe, fool, foam, loaf; /ie/ Faye, fail, chafe, defame; /ɑu/ Faust, fountain; /ɔi/ foil, typhoid; /ɪ/ fit, if, fin, fist; /ɛ/ fed, unfed, fetter, deaf; /æ/ fat, fad, calf, taffy; /ʊ/ foot, afoot, roof; /ʌ/ fun, puff, muffin, rough; /ə/ fatigue, elephant, buffoon, muffin; /ɝ/ fern, furs, first, unfurl; /ɚ/ offer, rougher, tougher, suffer. *Phrases:* Fern laughed after falling. Faye fed the fat fox. The fighters were fatigued after their defeat.

/v/ (*v*an)

/ɑ/ vomit, guava, avant; /u/ voodoo, moving, prove; /i/ veto, even, heave, peeved; /ɑu/ vow, vowel, avow; /ɑi/ vie, revive, hive, diving; /iu/ view, review, overview; /ou/ vote, revoke, vogue, cove; /ei/ vain, wave, David, vail; /ɑu/ vow, vowel; /ɔi/ voile, void, avoid; /ɪ/ give, vim, vigor, giving; /ɛ/ vent, Beverly, heavy, leaven; /æ/ vat, vamp, have, having; /ʊ/ hooves; /ʌ/ above, oven, hover; /ə/ avowal, heaven, oven; /ɝ/ verve, Verner, curve, serve; /ɚ/ over, rover, cover, Dover. *Phrases:* Vernon overrode the veto. Beverly covered the vat. Avoid giving Vi the scarves.

[1-8] *Ibid.* (see p. 79).

Stimulation Unit 25

Phonetic Symbol and Representative Word: /θ, ð/ (*th*in, *th*is)

Symbol Systems

International Phonetic Alphabet:/θ, ð/
Webster's New College Dictionary (1965): th, t̲h̲
Thorndike-Barnhardt Comprehensive Dictionary (1951): th[1], ŦH[2]
Northampton Charts (Yale, 1946): th, ŧh

Topographical Relationships of Phoneme Production

/θ/ (*th*in)	voiceless	lingua-dental	fricative	continuant
/ð/ (*th*is)	voiced	lingua-dental	fricative	continuant

MANDIBLE:
slightly lowered

LIPS:
unrounded

TONGUE:
Tip—in contact with lower posterior edge of upper incisors
Sides—in contact with upper molars

AIRSTREAM:
forced through small aperture between upper incisors and tongue tip, thus causing friction

NASAL PORT:
closed

VOCAL FOLDS:
/θ/ not vibrating; /ð/ vibrating

Stimulation Procedures

VISUAL-AUDITORY MODEL. A model demonstration is provided by the manipulation of the stimulator's face while the respondent observes. An auditory stimulus is usually given simultaneously as the stimulator is saying: "We are going to say /θ/ (*th*in) or /ð/ (*th*is)." This step may be repeated.

STARTING POSITION. Respondent's articulators should be in the starting position before the manipulation is initiated: lips parted; mandible lowered slightly from position of closure; tongue in customary, relaxed position; vocal folds not vibrating.

SIMULTANEOUS STIMULATION. Stimulator places fingers in position on respondent's face. As the manipulation takes place, the respondent may observe the stimulator's face and/or hear an auditory stimulus.

EXTRAORAL MANIPULATION /θ/ (*th*in)

1. Assume starting position.
2. Press index finger of each hand along upper lip and lower lip lines between points 3.
3. Airstream should be directed through lingua-dental opening.
4. Phonate for /ð/ (*th*is).

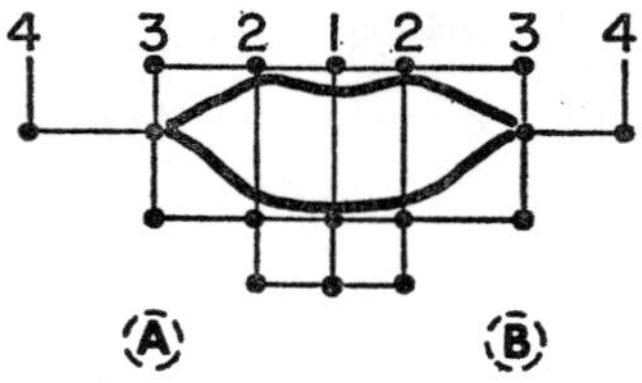

MANIPULATION MODEL: LIPS FORMAT.

EXTRAORAL MANIPULATION /ð/ (*th*is)

1. Assume starting position.
2. Firmly press index finger of one hand in a curved position along upper lip line between points 3; hold for slightly greater duration than for the /θ/ (*th*in).
3. Airstream should be directed through lingua-dental opening.
4. Phonate. (The stimulator may signal phonation by placing little finger against respondent's larynx.)

Stimulating /ɑ/ (c*a*lm, l*o*t) after the /θ, ð/ (*th*in, *th*is) provides an effective sound combination.

/θ, ð/ (*th*in, *th*is) Response Analysis and Extraoral Cues

AIRSTREAM. If initiation of airstream is a problem, use one hand to press gently but firmly at a point just below sternum. This pressure should generate a steady flow of air.

A strip of paper or a feather may be used to demonstrate the desired amount of airflow.

TONGUE. Although the protrusion of the tongue is sometimes exaggerated while establishing the position of the articulators, this exaggeration should not continue once the phoneme is stabilized.

VOCAL FOLDS. A finger may be placed on the respondent's larynx to signal phonation for /ð/ (*th*is).

/θ, ð/ (*th*in, *th*is) SELECTED PHONEME CHARACTERISTICS

DEVELOPMENTAL AGE:[1]

/θ/ th-, -th-, -th, -nt th, -rth = 6 yrs.; thr- = 7 yrs.; /ð/ ~~th~~, ~~thr~~-, = 6 yrs.; ~~th~~-, -~~thr~~ = 6 yrs.; -~~th~~-, -~~th~~ = 7 yrs.

FREQUENCY OF OCCURRENCE OF PHONEME:[2]

/θ/ 0.81%; thirty-fourth in order of occurrence. /ð/ 3.62%; eighth in order of occurrence.

VISUAL INTELLIGIBILITY:[3]

/θ/ not given; /ð/ 71% to 100%; composite 81%

VISUAL CONFUSION:[4]

/θ, ð/ (*th*in, *th*is)

AUDITORY INTELLIGIBILITY IN MILD-TO-SEVERE HEARING IMPAIRMENTS:[5]

/θ/ 52%; /ð/ 65%

AUDITORY CONFUSION:[6]

/ʃ, s, f, θ, tʃ/ (*sh*oe, *s*o, *f*ace, *th*in, *ch*in); /ʒ, z, v, ð, dʒ, j/ (a*z*ure, *z*one, *v*an, *th*is, *j*am, *y*et)

RELATIVE PHONETIC POWER:[7]

/θ/ 1; /ð/ 11 (range of 1 to 680)

PHONEMIC CONFUSION:[8]

/θ/ (*th*in), /f/ (*f*ace), /s/ (*s*o), /t/ (*t*o); /ð/ (*th*is), /v/ (*v*an), /z/ (*z*one), /d/ (*d*o)

TYPICAL SPELLING:

/θ/ *th* (*th*ink), *the* (absin*the*); /ð/ *th* (*th*is), *the* (ba*the*)

/θ, ð/ (*th*in, *th*is) PRACTICE MATERIALS

The sounds to be stimulated are /θ, ð/ (*th*in, *th*is). Only those words and phrases in which the respondent can articulate all of the sounds correctly, except the target phoneme, should be utilized for practice. The same stipulation applies to the practice materials provided at the end of this Section.

/θ/ (*th*in)

/θ/ bath, bathtub, menthol, Goths; /u/ booth, tooth, soothsayer; /i/ theme, teeth, thief, theater; /ɑu/ mouth; /ɑi/ thigh, python, writhe; /ju/ youth: /ou/ oath, both, loathsome; /ei/ faith, thane, eighth; /ɔ/ thong, moth, warmth; /ɪ/ thin, thick, myth, think; /ɛ/ theft, death, ethnic, Ethel; /æ/ bath, bathtub, thank, athlete; /ʌ/ thumb, doth, nothing; /ɝ/ third, birth, mirth, thirst. *Phrases:* The moth sought the warmth. The thin youth was eighth in line. Ethel thought the youth was thirsty.

/ð/ (*th*is)

/ð/ moths, broths, clothes, bother; /u/ youths, truths, smoothed, soothed; /i/ the, teethe, teething, wreaths; /ɑu/ thou, mouths, mouthing; /ɑi/ thy, tithe, tithing, writhed; /ou/ though, oaths, clothes; /ei/ they, bathe, bathing; /ɪ/ with, without; /ɛ/ them, then; /æ/ that,

[1-8] *Ibid.* (see p. 79).

fathom, paths, baths; /ʌ/ other, another; /ə/ heathen; /ɚ/ mother, bother, brother, other. *Phrases:* These babies teethed without pain. They bathed themselves. The mothers made wreaths.

COMPARATIVE PRACTICE MATERIALS

SECTION G: FRICATIVES (PART ONE)

The sounds to be stimulated are /h, f, v, θ, ð/ (*h*at, *f*ace, *v*an, *th*in, *th*is). Only those words and phrases in which the respondent can articulate all of the sounds correctly, except the target phoneme, should be utilized for practice.

	/h/ (*h*at)	/f/ (*f*ace)	/v/ (*v*an)	/θ/ (*th*in)	/ð/ (*th*is)
INITIAL POSITION:	hat	fat	vat		that
	hen	fen			then
		fan	van		than
		fin		thin	
		half	have		
	hair	fair			there
FINAL POSITION:		safe	save	bath	
			rave	wraith	

SECTION H: FRICATIVES AND AFFRICATES (PART TWO)

Representative Words:	*s*o	*z*one	*sh*oe	a*z*ure	*ch*in	*j*am
International Phonetic Alphabet:	/s/	/z/	/ʃ/	/ʒ/	/tʃ/	/dʒ/
Webster's New Collegiate Dictionary (1965):	s	z	sh	zh	ch	j
Thorndike-Barnhardt Comprehensive Dictionary (1951):	s	z	sh	zh	ch	j
Northampton Charts (Yale, 1946):	s	z	sh	zh	ch	j

The two pairs of voiced and voiceless fricatives, /s-z, ʃ-ʒ/ (*s*o, *z*one, *sh*oe, a*z*ure) and the voiced-voiceless pair of affricates /tʃ-dʒ/ (*ch*in, *j*am) continue the articulatory movement from a more forward position to a more backed position in the mouth. The /s-z, ʃ-ʒ/ (*s*o, *z*one, *sh*oe, a*z*ure) belong to the sibilant family of sounds and are often distorted. The resonance of /ʃ-ʒ/ (*sh*oe, a*z*ure) changes because of the protruding lip position.

The affricates /tʃ-dʒ/ (*ch*in, *j*am) are formed by a retracted /t-d/

(*to*, *do*) combined with a fronted /ʃ-ʒ/ (*sh*oe, a*z*ure). The rapid blending gives the auditory effect of one sound.

Stimulation Unit 26

Phonetic Symbol and Representative Word: /s, z/ (*s*o, *z*one)

Symbol Systems

International Phonetic Alphabet: /s, z/
Webster's New Collegiate Dictionary (1965): s, z
Thorndike-Barnhardt Comprehensive Dictionary (1951): s, z
Northampton Charts (Yale, 1946): s, z

Topographical Relationships of Phoneme Production

/s/ (*s*o)	voiceless	lingua-alveolar	fricative	continuant
/z/ (*z*one)	voiced	lingua-alveolar	fricative	continuant

MANDIBLE:
slightly lowered
LIPS:
neutral position
TONGUE:
Tip—raised to position back of upper incisors without making contact
Body—forms groove, makes contact with upper molars
AIRSTREAM:
forced through small aperture between tongue tip and incisors, thus causing friction
NASAL PORT:
closed
VOCAL FOLDS:
/s/ not vibrating; /z/ vibrating

Stimulation Procedures

VISUAL-AUDITORY MODEL. A model demonstration is provided by the manipulation of the stimulator's face while the respondent observes. An auditory stimulus is usually given simultaneously as the stimulator is saying: "We are going to say /s/ (*s*o) or /z/ (*z*one)." This step may be repeated.

STARTING POSITION. Respondent's articulators should be in the starting position before the manipulation is initiated: lips parted, mandible lowered slightly from position of closure, tongue in customary, relaxed position, vocal folds not vibrating.

SIMULTANEOUS STIMULATION. Stimulator places fingers in position on respondent's face. As the manipulation takes place, the respondent may observe the stimulator's face and/or hear an auditory stimulus.

EXTRAORAL MANIPULATION /s/ (*s*o)

1. Assume starting position.
2. Press thumb and third finger on upper lip points 2, directing the lips slightly toward upper lip points 3.
3. Initiate airstream for production of fricative sound.
4. Emit airstream through lingua-alveolar aperture.

EXTRAORAL MANIPULATION /z/ (*z*one)

1. Assume starting position.
2. Press thumb and third finger on upper lip points 2, directing the lips slightly toward upper lip points 3.
3. Initiate airstream for production of fricative sound.
4. Press firmly and with slightly greater duration than for the /s/ (*s*o).
5. Phonate. (The stimulator may signal phonation by placing little finger against respondent's larynx.)

If the above manipulations are not sufficient, use the additional manipulation procedures.

ADDITIONAL MANIPULATION

If the above stimulation does not produce the /s/ (*s*o) or /z/ (*z*one) sounds immediately, initiate a short series of oscillations of the thumb and third finger on upper lip points 2, as the auditory and/or visual stimuli are presented.

If the respondent prefers the tongue tip placed behind the lower incisors in the production of the /s/ (*s*o) and /z/ (*z*one) sounds, place the thumb and third finger on lower lip points 2. The same oscillation as above can be utilized.

If the respondent displays an "edge-to-edge" bite instead of a normal closure, even when a normal occlusion exists, suggest a chewing motion. When possible, stop the mandible in a moment of correct closure, thus illustrating to the respondent the position desired.

/s, z/ (*s*o, *z*one) Response Analysis and Extraoral Cues

AIRSTREAM. If the initiation of airstream is a problem, use one hand to press gently but firmly at a point above waistline and below juncture of ribs. This pressure should generate a steady flow of air. A strip of paper or feather may be used to demonstrate amount of air flow.

Tongue. If the sound produced is not sharp enough, the stimulation of pressing firmly with thumb and third finger between upper lip points 2 and 3 tends to bring sides of tongue into contact with molars and usually helps to eliminate breathiness. Firm pressure on lip points 2 (upper or lower points, depending upon desired tongue position) tends to stimulate a narrow groove in tongue body and to produce a sharper sound.

If the tongue and other articulatory movements are not properly executed, the /s, z/ (so, zone) may take the form of a bilateral or unilateral lisp.

In the normal position, the tongue makes contact with the upper teeth at the level of the incisors while the center forms a groove. The tongue tip is slightly lowered from the alveolar ridge. The friction is caused from forcing the air through the small aperture. If this process is reversed, causing the tongue tip to remain in contact with the alveolar ridge while one or both sides of the tongue lose contact with the upper teeth, the result is a bilateral or unilateral lisp. The resultant sound is a frictionalized /l/ which is not a regular phoneme in English.

If there is undue protrusion of the tongue, the resultant sounds will be /θ-ð/ (*th*in, *th*is), causing *sue* to become /θu/ and zoo to become /ðu/. If too much pressure is exerted behind the tongue tip, a whistling sound results.

Vocal Folds. A finger may be placed on the respondent's larynx to signal phonation for /z/ (*z*one).

/s, z/ (*s*o, *z*one) PHONODENTAL GUIDES

Chapter 5 gives details concerning preparation and placement of phonodental guides. Figures 5 and 6 in Chapter 5 illustrate the approximate points of lingual contact for the guides.

Phonodental guides and intraoral cues may be used independently or in combination with the extraoral manipulations.

The extraoral manipulation is usually effective for eliciting this phoneme, and intraoral stimulation is not required. If intraoral stimulation is needed, one or more of the following phonodental guides may be utilized.

Dental Floss Guides /s, z/ (*s*o, *z*one)

Raise tongue tip: two knotted dental floss guides placed between Maxillary Lateral Incisors and Cuspids (12-13 and 22-23).

Lower tongue tip: two knotted dental floss guides placed between Mandibular Central Incisors and Lateral Incisors (31-32 and 41-42).

Stemmed Wire Guides /s, z/ (*s*o, *z*one)

Raise tongue tip: longer stem of double-ended wire guides used to position tongue tip at alveolar ridge near Maxillary Lateral Incisors and Cuspids (12-13 and 22-23).

Lower tongue tip: shorter stem of double-ended wire guide used to position tongue tip behind Mandibular Central Incisors and Lateral Incisors (31-32 and 41-42).

Cue Sticks /s, z/ (*s*o, *z*one)

Cotton-tipped sticks dipped in cold water or parts of tongue depressors may be used to stimulate the same points for lingual contact as those given above.

/s, z/ (so, zone) SELECTED PHONEME CHARACTERISTICS

DEVELOPMENTAL AGE:[1]

/s/ -s-, -ks, -sm = 3.5 yrs.; s-, sk-, sm-, sn-, sp-, st-, -mps = 4 yrs.; -s = 4.5 yrs.; str- = 5 yrs.; -sl, skw-, -str, -rst = 6 yrs.; sl-, sw-, -sk, -st, skr-, spl-, spr-, -skr, -kst = 7 yrs.; -sp = 8 yrs.; /z/ -z- = 3.5 yrs.; z-, -z, -zm = 7 yrs.

FREQUENCY OF OCCURRENCE OF PHONEME:[2]

/s/ 3.74%; sixth in order of occurrence

/z/ 2.13%; seventeenth in order of occurrence

VISUAL INTELLIGIBILITY:[3]

/s/ 30% to 70%; composite 50%

/z/ 13% to 50%; composite 42%

VISUAL CONFUSION:[4]

/s, z, ʒ, t, dʒ, j/ (*s*o, *z*one, a*z*ure, *t*o, *j*am, *y*et)

AUDITORY INTELLIGIBILITY IN MILD-TO-SEVERE HEARING IMPAIRMENTS:[5]

/s/ 42%;

/z/ 51%

AUDITORY CONFUSION:[6]

/ʃ, s, f, θ, tʃ/ (*sh*oe, *s*o, *f*ace, *th*in, *ch*in)

/ʒ, z, v, ð, dʒ/ (a*z*ure, *z*one, *v*an, *th*is, *j*am)

RELATIVE PHONETIC POWER:[7]

/s/ 16; /z/ 16 (range of 1 to 680)

PHONEMIC CONFUSION:[8]

/s/ (*s*o), /t/ (*t*o), /θ/ (*th*in); /f/ (*f*ace);

/z/ (*z*one); /d/ (*d*o); /ð/ (*th*is); /v/ (*v*an)

TYPICAL SPELLING:

/s/ *c* (*c*ent); *ce* (dan*ce*); *ps* (*ps*alm); *s* (*s*o); *sc* (a*sc*end); *sch*

[1-8] *Ibid.* (see p. 79).

(*sch*ism); *sce* (acquie*sce*); *se* (moo*se*); *ss* (pa*ss*ing); *st* (fa*st*en); *sw* (an*sw*er); /z/ *cz* (*cz*ar); *es* (liv*es*); *s* (a*s*); *sc* (di*sc*ern); *se* (ro*se*); *ss* (sci*ss*ors); *z* (*z*oo); *ze* (do*ze*); *zz* (bu*zz*)

/s, z/ (*s*o, *z*one) PRACTICE MATERIALS

The sounds to be stimulated are /s/ (*s*o) and /z/ (*z*one). Only those words and phrases in which the respondent can articulate all of the sounds correctly, except the target phoneme, should be utilized for practice. The same stipulation applies to the practice materials provided at the end of this Section.

/s/ (*s*o)

/s/ (*s*o) /ɑ/ psalm, boss, sauce, sonnet; /u/ Sue, moose, loosen, ruse; /i/ see, cease, seat, descent; /ɑu/ sow, mouse, house, sound; /ɑi/ sigh, ice, sight, bison; /ju, iu/ suit, obtuse, Tuesday; /ou/ sow, dose, soul, soar; /ei/ say, ace, save, Mason; /ɔ/ saw, sought, song, boss; /ɔi/ soy, oyster, soil, voice; /ɪ/ sit, sip, miss, listen; /ɛ/ set, sell, less, guest; /æ/ sat, gas, salve, mass; /ʊ/ soot, puss, pussy; /ʌ/ sudden, sum, bus, muscle; /ə/ misses; /ɝ/ certain, burst, curse, sir; /ɚ/ Unser, presser, precursor, professor. *Phrases:* The mouse sniffed the cheese. Sip the soda. Sue likes the story of *Puss and Boots.*

/z/ (*z*one)

/z/ (*z*one) /ɑ/ Oz, cause, vase, nozzle; /u/ zoo, ooze, lose, bazooka; /i/ Zee, zeal, tease, weasel; /ɑu/ houses, vows, zounds, housing; /ɑi/ eyes, Zion, advise, design; /ju, ku/ use, fuse, amuse, clues; /ou/ ozone, rose, hose, posy; /ɔi/ toys, noise, poison, boys; /ɪ/ his, drizzle, fizz, dizzy; /ʊ/ bosom; /ʌ/ buzz, fuzzy, buzzard; /ə/ Zenobia, feasible, reasonable, pheasant; /ɝ/ furs, Xerxes, burrs; /ɚ/ Windsor, miser, laser, razor. *Phrases:* The Wizard of Oz has awed many boys. The teachers amaze the boys. Zach teases girls with bugs.

Stimulation Unit 27

Phonetic Symbol and Representative Word: /ʃ, ʒ/ (*sh*oe, a*z*ure)

Symbol Systems

International Phonetic Alphabet: /ʃ, ʒ/
Webster's New Collegiate Dictionary (1965): sh, zh
Thorndike-Barnhardt Comprehensive Dictionary (1951): sh, zh
Northampton Charts (Yale, 1946): sh, zh

Topographical Relationships of Phoneme Production

/ʃ/ voiceless lingua-palatal fricative
/ʒ/ voiced lingua-palatal fricative

MANDIBLE:
slightly lowered

LIPS:
protruded in round or oval shape

TONGUE:
Tip—directed upward toward alveolar ridge
Body—forms groove
Sides—in contact with maxillary teeth as far forward as premolars

AIRSTREAM:
emitted through opening between tongue tip and palate just posterior to alveolar ridge

NASAL PORT:
closed

VOCAL FOLDS:
/ʃ/ not vibrating; /ʒ/ vibrating

Stimulation Procedures

VISUAL-AUDITORY MODEL. A model demonstration is provided by the manipulation of the stimulator's face while the respondent observes. An auditory stimulus is usually given simultaneously as the stimulator is saying: "We are going to say /ʃ/ (*sh*oe) or /ʒ/ (a*z*ure)." This step may be repeated.

STARTING POSITION. Respondent's articulators should be in the starting position before the manipulation is initiated: lips parted; mandible lowered slightly from position of closure; tongue in customary, relaxed position; vocal folds not vibrating.

SIMULTANEOUS STIMULATION. Stimulator places fingers in position on respondent's face. As the manipulation takes place, the respondent may observe the stimulator's face and/or hear an auditory stimulus.

EXTRAORAL MANIPULATION /ʃ/ (*sh*oe)

1. Assume starting position.
2. Press thumb and third finger of one hand on upper lip points 3.
3. Press thumb and third finger of other hand on lower lip points 3.
4. Move fingers of both hands slightly toward the mid-lip line in order to form an elongated, scoop-like shape.
5. Initiate the airstream producing friction.
6. Emit airstream through lingua-alveolar aperture.

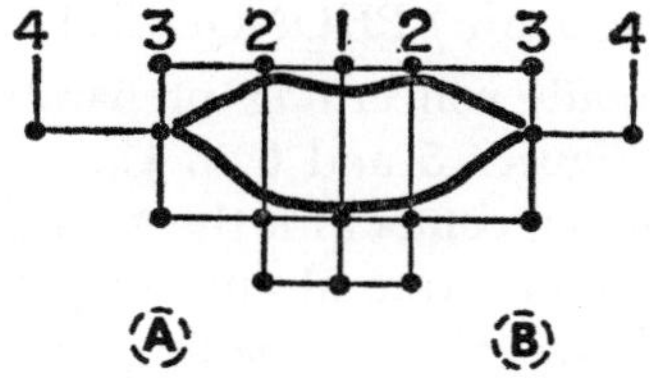

MANIPULATION MODEL: LIPS FORMAT.

EXTRAORAL MANIPULATION /ʒ/ (azure)

1. Assume starting position.
2. Press thumb and third finger of one hand on upper lip points 3.
3. Press thumb and third finger of other hand on lower lip points 3.
4. Move fingers of both hands slightly toward the mid-lip line in order to form an elongated, scoop-like shape.
5. Initiate the airstream producing friction.
6. Press firmly and with slightly greater duration than for the /ʃ/ (*sh*oe).
7. Phonate. (The stimulator may signal phonation by placing little finger against respondent's larynx.)

If the above manipulation is not sufficient, use the additional procedures.

ADDITIONAL MANIPULATION

1. If /ʃ/ (*sh*oe) or /ʒ/ (a*z*ure) is not produced satisfactorily after the above manipulation, grasp the cheeks between the thumb and the flat sides of the fingers at mid-lip line points 4 and move the lips toward the midline sufficiently to shape the lips in a scoop-like protrusion.
2. Another manipulation combines pressure of one hand on upper lip points 3 and of the other hand on lower lip points 3 with a slight movement by both hands toward the mid-lip line in order to form an elongated scoop-like shape.

/ʃ, ʒ/ (*sh*oe, a*z*ure) Response Analysis and Extraoral Cues

LIPS. The resonance changes for /ʃ/ (*sh*oe) and /ʒ/ (a*z*ure) because of lip protrusion.

AIRSTREAM. If the initiation of the airstream is a problem, use one hand to press gently but firmly at a point below the sternum.

VOCAL FOLDS. Slightly greater pressure of slightly longer duration than for /ʃ/ (*sh*oe) tends to bring about the voicing needed for /ʒ/ (a*z*ure).

A finger may be placed against the respondent's larynx to signal phonation.

/ʃ, ʒ/ (*sh*oe, a*z*ure) PHONODENTAL GUIDES

Chapter 5 gives details concerning preparation and placement of phonodental guides. Figures 5 and 6 in Chapter 5 illustrate the approximate points of lingual contact for the guides.

Phonodental guides and intraoral cues may be used independently or in combination with the extraoral manipulations.

The extraoral manipulation is usually effective for eliciting this phoneme, and intraoral stimulation is not required. If intraoral stimulation is needed, one or more of the following phonodental guides may be utilized.

Denture Guides /ʃ, ʒ/ (*sh*oe, a*z*ure)

Raise tongue sides: two denture guides placed between Maxillary Second Bicuspids and First Molars (15-16 and 25-26).

Dental Floss Guides /ʃ, ʒ/ (*sh*oe, a*z*ure)

Raise tongue sides: two knotted dental floss guides placed between Maxillary Second Bicuspids and First Molars (15-16 and 25-26).

Stemmed Wire Guides /ʃ, ʒ/ (*sh*oe, a*z*ure)

Raise tongue sides: tips of forked stemmed wire guide adjusted so tips touch alveolar ridge in approximate area of Maxillary Second Bicuspids and First Molars (15-16 and 25-26); single long stemmed wire guide used to raise tongue or to indicate contact areas.

Cue Sticks /ʃ, ʒ/ (*sh*oe, a*z*ure)

Cotton-tipped sticks dipped in cold water or parts of tongue depressors may be used to stimulate the same points for lingual contact as those given above.

/ʃ, ʒ/ (*sh*oe, a*z*ure) SELECTED PHONEME CHARACTERISTICS

DEVELOPMENTAL AGE:[1]

/ʃ/ sh-, -sh = 4 yrs.; -sh- = 4.5 yrs; -shr = 5 yrs.; shr- = 7 yrs.; /ʒ/ -zh-, -zh = 7 yrs.

FREQUENCY OF OCCURRENCE OF PHONEME:[2]

/ʃ/ 0.49%; thirty-sixth in order of occurrence

/ʒ/ 0.00%; forty-second in order of occurrence

VISUAL INTELLIGIBILITY:[3]

/ʃ/ 32% to 76%; composite 58%, /ʒ/ not given

VISUAL CONFUSION:[4]

/s, z, ʒ, t, dʒ, j/ (*s*o, *z*one, a*z*ure, *t*o, *j*am, *y*et)

AUDITORY INTELLIGIBILITY IN MILD-TO-SEVERE HEARING IMPAIRMENTS:[5]

/ʃ/ 37%; /ʒ/ not given

AUDITORY CONFUSION:[6]

/ʃ, s, f, θ, tʃ/ (*sh*oe, *s*o, *f*ace, *th*in, *ch*in)

/ʒ, z, v, dʒ, j/ (a*z*ure, *z*one, *v*an, *j*am, *y*et)

RELATIVE PHONETIC POWER:[7]

/ʃ/ 80; /ʒ/ 20 (range of 1 to 680)

PHONEMIC CONFUSION:[8]

/ʃ/ (*sh*oe), /tʃ/ (*ch*in), /s/ (*s*o); /ʒ/ (a*z*ure), /dʒ/ (*j*am), /z/ (*z*one)

TYPICAL SPELLING:

/ʃ/ *c* (spe*c*ial); *ce* (o*ce*an); *ch* (ma*ch*ine); *ci* (fa*ci*al); *che* (mousta*che*); *psh* (*psh*aw); *s* (*s*ure); *sci* (con*sci*ous); *sch* (*sch*ist); *se* (nau*se*ous); *sh* (*sh*ow); *si* (pen*si*on); *ss* (ti*ss*ue); *ssi* (mi*ssi*on); *ti* (sta*ti*on); *x* (lu*x*ury); /ʒ/ *z* (a*z*ure); *zi* (gla*zi*er); *s* (plea*s*ure); *si* (vi*si*on); *ssi* (absci*ssi*on); g (re-gime); *j* (*j*abot)

/ʃ, ʒ/ (*sh*oe, a*z*ure) PRACTICE MATERIALS

The sounds to be stimulated are /ʃ/ (*sh*oe) and /ʒ/ (a*z*ure). Only those words and phrases in which the respondent can articulate all of the sounds correctly, except for the target phoneme, should be utilized for practice. The same stipulation applies to the practice materials provided at the end of this Section.

/ʃ/ (*sh*oe)

/ɑ/ shot, wash, Henshaw; /u/ tissue, shoe, cashew; /i/ she, machine, sheet, hashish; /ɑu/ shout, shower; /ɑi/ shine, shoeshine, shy; /iu/ issue, tissue; /ou/ ocean, social, quotient, chauffeur; /ei/ gracious, nation, station; /ɔ/ Shaw, wash, caution; /ɪ/ dish, wished, Chicago; /ɛ/ transgression, chef, shed, mesh; /æ/ shall, shack, mash, passion; /ʊ/ sure, censure, sugar, shook; /ʌ/ luxury, shut, mush, gushing; /ə/ conscious, tension, mansion; /ɝ/ shirk, shirt, Hirsch, Hershey; /ɚ/ fissure. *Phrases:* She washed the dishes. Shaw lived in luxury. The chef measured the sugar.

/ʒ/ (a*z*ure)

/ɑ/ massage, garage, barrage; /u/ rouge; /i/ negligee, adhesion; /iu/ Bijou; /ei/ beige, occasion, Asia; /ɪ/ vision; /ʌ/ jabot; /ə/ vision; /ɚ/ leisure, pleasure, measure, lesion. *Phrases:* Can you envision a trip to Asia? The beige car was parked in the garage. It is a pleasure to have a massage.

[1-8] *Ibid.* (see p. 79).

Stimulation Unit 28

Phonetic Symbol and Representative Word: /tʃ, dʒ/ (*ch*in, *j*am)

Symbol Systems

International Phonetic Alphabet:/tʃ, dʒ/
Webster's New Collegiate Dictionary (1965): ch, j
Thorndike-Barnhardt Comprehensive Dictionary (1951): ch, j
Northampton Charts (Yale, 1946): ch, j

Topographical Relationships of Phoneme Production
/tʃ/ voiceless lingua-palatal affricate
/dʒ/ voiced lingua-palatal affricate

MANDIBLE:
slightly lowered
LIPS:
slightly more rounded than for the /t/ (*t*o) and /d/ (*d*o)
TONGUE:
Tip—slightly more retracted than for /ʃ, ʒ/ (*sh*oe, a*z*ure). The emission of retracted /t, d/ quickly blends with /ʃ, ʒ/ so that the result gives the auditory effect of one continuous sound /tʃ, dʒ/ (*ch*in) and (*j*am).
Body—forms groove as sound is emitted
SIDES:
in contact with maxillary teeth as far forward as premolars.
AIRSTREAM:
emitted through small opening between tongue tip and post-alveolar ridge
NASAL PORT:
closed
VOCAL FOLDS:
/tʃ/ not vibrating; /dʒ/ vibrating

Stimulation Procedures

VISUAL-AUDITORY MODEL. A model demonstration is provided by the manipulation of the stimulator's face while the respondent observes. An auditory stimulus is usually given simultaneously as the stimulator is saying: "We are going to say /tʃ/ (*ch*in) or /dʒ/ (*j*am)." This step may be repeated.

STARTING POSITION. Respondent's articulators should be in the starting position before the manipulation is initiated: lips parted; mandible lowered slightly from position of closure; tongue in customary, relaxed position; vocal folds not vibrating.

Simultaneous Stimulation. Stimulator places fingers in position on respondent's face. As the manipulation takes place, the respondent may observe the stimulator's face and/or hear an auditory stimulus.

EXTRAORAL MANIPULATION /tʃ/ (*ch*in)

1. Assume starting position.
2. Place index finger of one hand on upper lip point 1.
3. Exert slight pressure.
4. Remove finger with flicking motion.
5. Quickly press lower lip points 3 with thumb and third finger of the same hand.
6. Lower mandible sharply

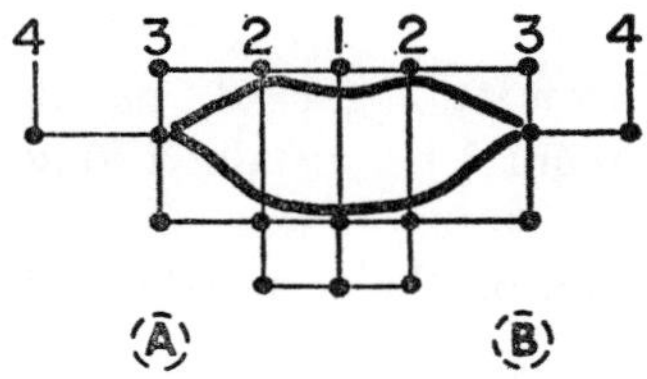

MANIPULATION MODEL: LIPS FORMAT.

EXTRAORAL MANIPULATION /dʒ/ (*j*am)

1. Assume starting position.
2. Place index finger of one hand on upper lip point 1.
3. Exert slight pressure.
4. Remove finger with flicking motion.
5. Quickly and firmly press lower lip points 3 with thumb and middle finger of the same hand. Hold for slightly greater duration than for /tʃ/ (*ch*in)
6. Lower mandible sharply to bring about a quick expulsion of air from the lungs, followed by air friction emitted through the lingua-alveolar aperture.
7. Phonate. (The stimulator may signal phonation by placing little finger against respondent's larynx.)

If the above manipulation is not sufficient, use the additional manipulation procedures.

ADDITIONAL MANIPULATION

1. After the stimulation for the /t, d/ elements of /tʃ/ (*ch*in) and /dʒ/ (*j*am), press the cheeks at mid-lip line points 4 between the thumb and the flat sides of the fingers and move the lips toward the mid-line in order to shape the lips into a scoop-like protrusion.

2. If the above is not successful, combine the pressure of one hand on upper lip points 3 and of the other hand on lower lip points 3 with a slight movement of both hands toward the mid-line in order to form an elongated, scoop-like shape.

/tʃ, dʒ/ (*ch*in, *j*am) Response Analysis and Extraoral Cues

The affricates /tʃ/ (*ch*in) /dʒ/ (*j*am) are formed by a retracted /t-d/ combining with /ʃ-ʒ/ in order to form the new sound. Emission of the retracted /t-d/ quickly blends with /ʃ-ʒ/ so that the result gives the auditory effect of one sound.

Tongue. The first part of the /tʃ/ (*ch*in) is a /t/ sound and is signaled but by a quick, light, flicking motion of the index finger.

Airstream. A strip of paper or feather may be used to demonstrate amount of air flow.

Vocal Folds. The stimulation for /d/ of /dʒ/ (*j*am) requires that pressure on upper lip point 1 be sustained long enough for phonation to be initiated.

A finger may be placed on the respondent's larynx to signal phonation.

/tʃ, dʒ/ (*ch*in, *j*am) PHONODENTAL GUIDES

The extraoral manipulation is usually effective for eliciting this phoneme, and intraoral stimulation is not required. If intraoral stimulation is needed, one or more of the following phonodental guides may be utilized.

Dental Floss Guides /tʃ, dʒ/ (*ch*in, *j*am)

Raise tongue sides: two knotted dental floss guides placed between Maxillary Cuspids and First Bicuspids (13-14 and 23-24).

Stemmed Wire Guides /tʃ, dʒ/ (*ch*in, *j*am)

Raise tongue sides: tips of forked stemmed wire guide adjusted so tips touch alveolar ridge in approximate area of Maxillary Cuspids and Bicuspids (13-14 and 23-24); single long stemmed wire guide used to raise tongue or to indicate contact areas.

Cue Sticks /tʃ, dʒ/ *ch*in, *j*am

Cotton-tipped sticks dipped in cold water or parts of tongue depressors may be used to stimulate the same points for lingual contact as those given above.

Note: The blending of the elements of this sound is not always easy; however, if the consonant sound in Stimulation Units 21 and 27 are learned, first through extra and/or intraoral stimulators, the suggested extraoral stimulation for /tʃ, dʒ/ (*ch*in, *j*am) usually produces the phoneme.

/tʃ, dʒ/ (*ch*in, *j*am) SELECTED PHONEME CHARACTERISTICS

DEVELOPMENTAL AGE:[1]

/tʃ/ ch-, -ch-, -ch = 4.5 yrs.; -rch = 6 yrs.; /dʒ/ j- = 4 yrs.; -j- = 5 yrs.; -rj = 6 yrs.; -j, -jd = 7 yrs.

FREQUENCY OF OCCURRENCE OF PHONEME:[2]

/tʃ/ 0.31%; thirty-seventh in order of occurrence
/dʒ/ 0.28%; thirty-ninth in order of occurrence

VISUAL INTELLIGIBILITY:[3]

/tʃ/ 15% to 40%; composite 45%;
/dʒ/ 31% to 40%; composite 48%

VISUAL CONFUSION:[4]

/s, z, ʒ, t, dʒ, j/ (*s*o, *z*one, a*z*ure, *t*o, *j*am, *y*et)

AUDITORY INTELLIGIBILITY IN MILD-TO-SEVERE HEARING IMPAIRMENTS:[5]

not given

AUDITORY CONFUSION:[6]

/ʃ, s, f, θ, tʃ/ (*sh*oe, *s*o, *f*ace, *th*in, *ch*in);
/ʒ, z, v, ð, dʒ, j/ (a*z*ure, *z*one, *v*an, *th*is, *j*am, *y*et)

RELATIVE PHONETIC POWER:[7]

/tʃ/ 42 /dʒ/ 23, (range 1 to 680)

PHONEMIC CONFUSION:[8]

/tʃ/ (*ch*in), /ʃ/ (*sh*oe), /t/ (*t*o), /ʔ/ (glottal stop);
/dʒ/ (*j*am), /ʒ/ (a*z*ure), /g/ (*g*o); /n/ (*n*o)

TYPICAL SPELLING:

/tʃ/ *ch* (*ch*air); *tch* (ma*tch*); *ti* (ques*ti*on); *te* (righ*te*ous); /t/ (fu*t*ure); /dʒ/ *j* (*j*oke); *g* (*g*erm); *gg* (exa*gg*erate); *gi* (reli*gi*on); *ge* (pi*ge*on); *d* (ver*d*ure); *di* (sol*di*er); *dg* (ju*dg*ment); *dge* (e*dge*)

/tʃ, dʒ (*ch*in, *j*am) PRACTICE MATERIALS

The sounds to be stimulated are /tʃ/ (*ch*in) and /dʒ/ (*j*am). Only those words and phrases in which the respondent can articulate all of the sounds correctly, except the target phoneme, should be utilized for practice. The same stipulation applies to the practice materials provided at the end of this Section.

/tʃ/ (*ch*in)

/ɑ/ watch, chock, watched; /u/ chew, mooch, moocher; /i/ teach, Medici, cheek, peaches; /ɑu/ chow, pouch, grouchy; /ɑi/ child,

[1-8] *Ibid.* (see p. 79).

righteous, chide; /ju, iu/ chew; /ou/ choke, poach, poached, broach; /ei/ chain, aitch, aitches; /ɔ/ chalk, watch; /ɔi/ Choy; /ɪ/ ditch, pitched, chick, itch; /ɛ/ chair, cello, check, etching; /æ/ catch, latch, match, patch; /ʊ/ Butch, butcher; /ʌ/ chum, chug, such, touch; /ə/ bachelor, question, righteous, pitcher; /ɝ/ church, perch, birch; /ɚ/ nature, furniture, perchance. *Phrases:* The butcher questioned the purchase. Teach the children to march. Butch choked on the chicken.

/dʒ/ (*j*am)

/ɑ/ lodge, logic, Joplin, John; /u/ juice, stooge, Jupiter, jute; /i/ Egypt, region, Jean, seige; /ɑu/ joust, gouge, gouging, jowl; /ɑi/ jibe, oblige, obliged; /ju, iu/ juice, Judas, June, Jew; /ou/ Joe, doze, logician, Joan; /ei/ cage, sage, jail, age; /ɔ/ jaw, forge; /ɔi/ joy, voyage, adjoin, overjoyed; /ɛ/ gem, ledger, wedge, edge; /æ/ jam, Jack, badge, Japan; /ʊ/ jury; /ʌ/ jump, judge, budge, jug; /ə/ legion, cordial, sandwiches, surgeon; /ɝ/ urge, surge, germ, adjourn; /ɚ/ soldier, lodgers, germane, badger. *Phrases:* Joe urged Joan to join Jack. The soldier joined the legion. The badger jumped out of the cage.

COMPARATIVE PRACTICE MATERIALS

SECTION H: FRICATIVES AND AFFRICATES (PART TWO)

The sounds to be stimulated are /s, z, ʃ, ʒ, tʃ, dʒ/ (*s*o, *z*one, *sh*oe, a*z*ure, *ch*in, and *j*am). Only those words and phrases in which the respondent can articulate all of the sounds correctly, except the target phoneme, should be utilized for practice.

	/s/ (*s*o)	/z/ (*z*one)	/ʃ/ (*sh*oe)	/ʒ/ (a*z*ure)	/tʃ/ (*ch*in)	/dʒ/ (*j*am)
INITIAL POSITION:	so	Zoe	show		choke	Joe
	seen	Zenith	sheen			Jean
	Sam		sham		champion	jam
	Sue	zoo	shoe		chew	Jew
FINAL POSITION:	ass	as	ash		aitch	
	ace	"A's"			"H"	age
	mass		mash		match	Madge

SECTION 1: FRICATIVES AND SEMIVOWELS

Representative words:	*what*	*we*	*let*	*rat*	*yet*
International Phonetic Alphabet:	hw	w	l	r	j
Webster's New Collegiate Dictionary (1965):	hw	w	l	r	y

Thorndike-Barnhardt Comprehensive Dictionary (1951):	hw	w	l	r	y
Northampton Charts (Yale, 1946):	wh	w-	l	r-	y-

The last group of consonant sounds to be used for stimulation includes the voiced fricative /w/ (*w*e); the voiceless fricative /hw/ (*wh*at), considered by many to be the voiceless analogue of /w/ (*w*e) when the *wh* is not pronounced as /w/ (*w*e); the voiced semivowel glide /l/ (*l*ook); the voiced semivowel /r/ (*r*at); and the voiced semivowel glide /j/ (*y*et). The point of articulation is the same for /w, hw/ (*w*e, *wh*at), however, the relationship of /l, r, j/ (*l*ook, *r*at, *y*et) is distant. The production of this group of sounds moves from a forward, visible position to a backed or invisible position. The fricatives /w, hw/ (*w*e, *wh*at) are bilabial sounds produced as the position of the following vowel sound is assumed.

The lingua-alveolar /l/ (*l*et) has the distinction of being the only English sound that is emitted laterally. In articulating the /l/ (*l*et), the lips and teeth play a relatively unimportant role. The tongue tip is placed on the alveolar ridge back of the upper incisors. The side or sides of the tongue are lowered allowing the airstream to be emitted laterally. The /s, z, (*s*o, *z*one) sounds are sometimes pronounced with the articulatory organs in the /l/ (*l*et) position, thus producing a lateral lisp.

The consonant /r/ (*r*at) is produced by placing the articulatory organs in approximately the reverse position for that of /l/ (*l*et). In articulating /r/ (*r*at), the sides of the tongue touch the maxillary teeth from back to just short of the incisors. The tongue tip is curved upward to a position back of the Maxillary Incisors.

The /r/ (*r*at) is an extremely variable sound and is subject to phonotactic influences. The /r/ (*r*at) has numerous allophones that are produced in similar positions. The treatment of these sounds constitutes one of the distinguishing characteristics of regional speech. The *r* in certain positions is a consonant, glide, or vowel. See the discussion of the vowel /ɝ/ (bi*r*d). Fundamentally different movements are required to produce the various allophones.

/j/ (*y*et) is a lingua-palatal, semivowel glide. A glide is a sound produced by an uninterrupted movement from the position of one sound to that of another. The teeth and lips play an unimportant role. The organs assume practically the same position as for the vowel /i/ (*b*e). As the sound is produced, it quickly assumes the articulatory position of the vowel which immediately follows as in *you* /ju/.

Stimulation Unit 29

Phonetic Symbol and Representative Word: /hw, w/ (*wh*at, *w*e)

Symbol Systems

International Phonetic Alphabet: /hw, w/
Webster's New Collegiate Dictionary (1965): hw, w
Thorndike-Barnhardt Comprehensive Dictionary (1951): hw, w
Northampton Charts (Yale, 1946): wh, w-

Topographical Relationships of Phoneme Production

/hw/ (*wh*at) voiceless bilabial glide
/w/ (*w*e) voiced bilabial semivowel glide

MANDIBLE:
at highest position to accommodate tongue

LIPS:
rounded

TONGUE:
Tip—touching back of lower front incisors
Back—raised and arched toward velum

AIRSTREAM:
emitted through narrow passage between tongue and velum

NASAL PORT:
closed

VOCAL FOLDS:
/hw/ not vibrating: /w/ vibrating

Stimulation Procedures

VISUAL-AUDITORY MODEL. A model demonstration is provided by the manipulation of the stimulator's face while the respondent observes. An auditory stimulus is usually given simultaneously as the stimulator is saying: "We are going to say /hw/ (*wh*at) or /w/ (*w*e)." This step may be repeated.

STARTING POSITION. Respondent's articulators should be in the starting position before the manipulation is initiated: lips parted; mandible lowered slightly from position of closure; tongue in customary, relaxed position; vocal folds not vibrating.

SIMULTANEOUS STIMULATION. Stimulator places fingers in position on respondent's face. As the manipulation takes place, the respondent may observe the stimulator's face and/or hear an auditory stimulus.

EXTRAORAL MANIPULATION /hw/ (*wh*at)

1. Assume starting position.
2. Place thumb and third finger of one hand on mid-lip points 3.

3. Move lips into the small rounded position of /u/ (b*oo*t).
4. Place other hand below the sternum, and press inward and upward with a sudden movement.
5. Release thumb and third finger of first hand as expelled air reaches oral cavity.

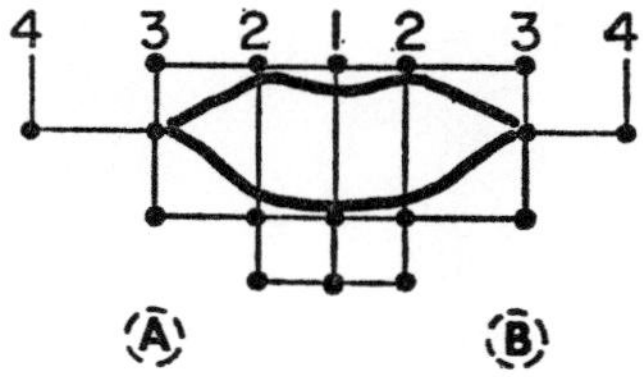

MANIPULATION MODEL: LIPS FORMAT.

EXTRAORAL MANIPULATION /w/ (*w*e)

1. Assume starting position.
2. Place thumb and third finger on mid-line points 3.
3. Move lips into the small rounded position of /u/ (b*oo*t).
4. Phonate as movement into the succeeding sound is initiated. (The stimulator may signal phonation by placing little finger against respondent's larynx.)

If the above manipulations are not sufficient, use the additional manipulation procedures.

ADDITIONAL MANIPULATION

1. The extreme vowels of /ɑ/ (c*a*lm, l*o*t) and /i/ (b*e*) may be combined with /hw/ (*wh*at) and /w/ (*w*e) in order to facilitate production through the sudden change in lip position for the succeeding sound.
2. Care should be taken not to press too hard when stimulating the airstream for the /hw/ (*wh*at).

/hw, w/ (*wh*at, *w*e) Response Analysis and Extraoral Cues

In some instances, respondents may have great difficulty in producing the /hw/ (*wh*at). One pronunciation is as acceptable as the other. Time should not be wasted on this distinction.

LIPS. A straw or pencil can be used to assist respondents in sensing the rounded position of the /u/ (b*oo*t), /hw/ (*wh*at), and /w/ (*w*e).

VOCAL FOLDS. A finger may be placed on the respondent's larynx to signal phonation for /w/ (*w*e).

/hw, w/ (*wh*at, *w*e) SELECTED PHONEME CHARACTERISTICS

DEVELOPMENTAL AGE:[1]

/hw/ hw-, -hw- = not produced correctly by 75 percent of the subjects by 8 years of age; /w/ w-, -w-, = 3 yrs.; tw-, kw- = 4 yrs.; skw- = 6 yrs.; sw- = 7 yrs.

FREQUENCY OF OCCURRENCE OF PHONEME:[2]

/hw/ 0.22%; fortieth in order of occurrence
/w/ 2.74%; thirteenth in order of occurrence

VISUAL INTELLIGIBILITY:[3]

/hw/ not given;
/w/ 70% to 100%; composite 73%

VISUAL CONFUSION:[4]

/p, w, hw/ (*p*at, *w*e, *wh*at)

AUDITORY INTELLIGIBILITY IN MILD-TO-SEVERE HEARING IMPAIRMENTS:[5]

/hw/ not given;
/w/ 78%

AUDITORY CONFUSION:[6]

/w, r, l/ (*w*e, *r*at, *l*et)

RELATIVE PHONETIC POWER:[7]

not given

PHONEMIC CONFUSION:[8]

/hw/ (*wh*at) /w/ (*w*e), /u/ (b*oo*t), /l/ (*l*et);
/w/ (*w*e) /hw/ (*wh*at), /h/ (*r*at), /ʊ/ (f*oo*t), /l/ (*l*et)

TYPICAL SPELLING:

/hw/ *wh* (*wh*at); /w/ *u* (q*u*ick); *w* (*w*ant); *u* (pers*u*ade); *o* (ch*o*ir); *qu* (*qu*ick); *gu* (*gu*ava)

/hw, w/ (*wh*at, *w*e) PRACTICE MATERIALS

The sounds to be stimulated are /hw/ (*wh*at) and /w/ (*w*e). Only those words and phrases in which the respondent can articulate all of the sounds correctly, except for the target phoneme, should be utilized for practice. The same stipulation applies to the practice materials provided at the end of this Section.

/hw/ (*wh*at)

/ɑ/ what; /u/ whoopee, whoop; /i/ wheel, wheeze, wheat; /ɑi/ why, while, white, whine; /ou/ whoa, nowhere; /ei/ whey, whale; /ɔ/ wharf; /ɪ/ whither, which, whim, whip; /ɛ/ whet, where, whether, when; /æ/ wham, whack; /ʊ/ whoopee, whooping; /ʌ/ what; /ɝ/ whir, whirl, awhirl. *Phrases:* What is the best wheat? Where is the white whale?

/w/ (*w*e)

/ɑ/ watt, wand, wander; /u/ woo, womb, wooer, woof; /i/ weal, wee, weeping, Peewee; /ɑu/ wow, pow-wow, wows; /ɑi/ wile, wine, wight,

[1-8] *Ibid.* (see p. 79).

wide; /ou/ woe, woke; /ei/ way, wail, waving, wailing; /ɔ/ warm, warden, Waugh, wort; /ɪ/ witch, wither, window, willow; /ɛ/ wear, wet, weather, wen; /æ/ wag, WAC; /ʊ/ woods, wolf, would, wool; /ʌ/ one-time, wonder; /ə/ away; /ɝ/ were, word, worm. *Phrases:* We wear lightweight wool. Warm weather is wonderful. The woods are wet. The willows waved in the wind.

Stimulation Unit 30

Phonetic Symbol and Representative Word: /l/ (*l*et)

Symbol Systems

International Phonetic Alphabet: /l/
Webster's New Collegiate Dictionary (1965): l
Thorndike-Barnhardt Comprehensive Dictionary (1951): l
Northampton Charts (Yale, 1946): l

Topographical Relationships of Phoneme Production

/l/ (*l*et) voiced lateral lingua-alveolar semivowel continuant

MANDIBLE:
slightly lowered
LIPS:
slightly rounded or normal
TONGUE:
Tip—touches alveolar ridge
Sides—lowered from contact with upper molars
AIRSTREAM:
emitted laterally in mouth cavity
NASAL PORT:
closed
VOCAL FOLDS:
vibrating

Stimulation Procedures

VISUAL-AUDITORY MODEL. A model demonstration is provided by the manipulation of the stimulator's face while the respondent observes. An auditory stimulus is usually given simultaneously with the stimulator saying: "We are going to say /l/ (*l*et)." This step may be repeated.

STARTING POSITION. Respondent's articulators should be in the starting position before the manipulation is initiated: lips parted; mandible lowered slightly from postion of closure; tongue in customary, relaxed position; vocal folds not vibrating.

SIMULTANEOUS STIMULATION. Stimulator places fingers in position on respondent's face. As the manipulation takes place, the respondent may observe the stimulator's face and/or hear an auditory stimulus.

EXTRAORAL MANIPULATION /l/ (*l*et)

1. Assume starting position.
2. Place thumb and middle finger in a flattened position on upper lip points 2.
3. Press evenly while phonating. (The stimulator may signal phonation by placing little finger against respondent's larynx.)

If the above manipulation is not sufficient, use the additional manipulation procedures.

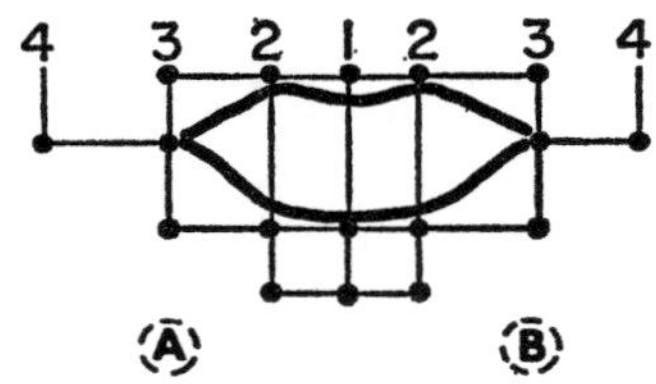

MANIPULATION MODEL: LIPS FORMAT.

ADDITIONAL MANIPULATION /l/ (*l*et)

1. When /w/ (*w*e) is substituted for /l/ (*l*et), place thumb and third finger in a flattened position between lip points 2-3.
2. Place thumb and middle finger on lower lip points 3 and hold lips in a slightly extended position in order to avoid rounding.

It is easier to teach /l/ (*l*et) as an initial sound as in *look, lame, let.* If the /l/ (*l*et) comes between two vowel sounds, teach it as an initial sound, e.g. "Billy" should be taught as "Bi/ly."

/l/ (*l*et) Response Analysis and Extraoral Cues

TONGUE. The tongue tip makes contact with the alveolar ridge above the Maxillary Incisors. The /l/ (*l*et), like most of the other sounds in English can be pulled forward or backed through the principle of phonotactics.

If the substitution of /w/ (*w*e) for /l/ (*l*et) persists, it may be that the tongue is not in contact with the alveolar ridge. A tongue depressor may be used to elevate the tongue and to indicate alveolar contact areas.

AIRSTREAM. The air is emitted through one or both sides of the tongue, depending upon the habit of the individual.

VOCAL FOLDS. A finger may be placed on the respondent's larynx to signal phonation.

/l/ (*l*et) PHONODENTAL GUIDES

Chapter 5 gives details concerning preparation and placement of phonodental guides. Figures 5 and 6 in Chapter 5 illustrate the approximate points of lingual contact for the guides.

Phonodental guides and intraoral cues may be used independently or in combination with the extraoral manipulations. If intraoral stimulation is needed, one or more of the following phonodental guides may be utilized.

Dental Floss Guides /l/ (*l*et)

Raise front of tongue: three knotted dental floss guides placed in the following manner: one between Maxillary Central Incisors (11-21) and two placed between Maxillary Cuspids and First Bicuspids (13-14 and 23-24).

Stemmed Wire Guides /l/ (*l*et)

Raise front of tongue: tips of forked stemmed wire guide adjusted so tips touch alveolar ridge in approximate area of Maxillary Cuspids and First Bicuspids (13-14 and 23-24); single long stemmed wire guide used to raise tongue or to indicate contact areas.

Cue Sticks /l/ (*l*et)

Cotton-tipped sticks dipped in cold water or parts of tongue depressors may be used to stimulate the same points for lingual contact as those given above.

/l/ (*l*et) SELECTED PHONEME CHARACTERISTICS

DEVELOPMENTAL AGE:[1]

l-, -l-, pl-, kl-, gl-, -lp, -lt = 4 yrs.; -lf = 4.5 yrs.; fl-, -lb = 5 yrs.; -l, -lk, -pl, -kl, -bl, -gl, -fl, -sl, -ngkl, -nggl = 6 yrs.; sl-, -lz, lth, spl- = 7 yrs.

FREQUENCY OF OCCURRENCE OF PHONEME:[2]

3.62%; seventh in order of occurrence

VISUAL INTELLIGIBILITY:[3]

30% to 90%; composite 58%

VISUAL CONFUSION:[4]

/t, d, n, l/ (*to, do, no, l*et)

AUDITORY INTELLIGIBILITY IN MILD-TO-SEVERE HEARING IMPAIRMENTS:[5]

87%

AUDITORY CONFUSION:[6]

/w, r, l/ (*w*e, *r*at, *l*et)

RELATIVE PHONETIC POWER:[7]

100 (range of 1 to 680)

PHONEMIC CONFUSION:[8]

/l/ (*l*et), /r/ (*r*at), /hw/ (*wh*at), /w/ (*w*e), /j/ (*y*et)

TYPICAL SPELLING:

l (*l*ate); *ll* (ho*ll*y); *le* (pa*le*); *sle* (i*sle*); *ln* (ki*ln*); *sl* (i*sl*and); *tle* (whis*tle*); *el* (nick*el*)

/l/ (*l*et) PRACTICE MATERIALS

The sound to be stimulated is /l/ (*l*et). Only those words and phrases in which the respondent can articulate all of the sounds correctly, except the target phoneme, should be substituted for practice. The same stipulation applies to the practice materials provided at the end of this Section.

/l/ (*l*et)

/ɑ/ lot, doll, hollow, log; /u/ loom, cool, foolish, loot; /i/ lead, feel, leap, peel; /au/ loud, towel, howling, allow; /ɑi/ live, mile, wily, Lyle; /ju/ yule; /ou/ load, hold, bowl, toll; /ei/ lame, daily, lake, lane; /ɔ/ log, call, vault, lawn; /ɔi/ loin, boil, boiling, toil; /ɪ/ live, linnet, linen; /ɛ/ leg, mellow, lemon, leopard; /æ/ lack, hallowed, lad, lamb; /ʊ/ look, full, bully, bullet; /ʌ/ love, dull, gully, gullet; /æ/ lamb, last, lamp, pal; /ɝ/ learn, alert, swirl; /ɚ/ antler, fuller, duller, curler. *Phrases:* The bully is bowling. Learn to keep alert. A hollow log mellows. Lyle toiled daily. Lucy boiled lemons.

Stimulation Unit 31

Phonetic Symbol and Representative Word: /r/ (*r*at)

Symbol Systems

International Phonetic Alphabet: /r/
Webster's New Collegiate Dictionary (1965): r
Thorndike-Barnhardt Comprehensive Dictionary (1951): r
Northampton Charts (Yale, 1946): r-

Topographical Relationships of Phoneme Production

/r/ (*r*at) voiced lingua-alveolar fricative semivowel continuant

MANDIBLE:

slightly lowered

LIPS:

rounded

TONGUE:

Tip—upward to position slightly back of alveolar ridge
Sides—in contact with upper molars

[1-8] *Ibid.* (see p. 79).

Airstream:
emitted through mouth
Nasal Port:
closed
Vocal Folds:
vibrating

Stimulation Procedures

Visual-Auditory Model. A model demonstration is provided by the manipulation of the stimulator's face while the respondent observes. An auditory stimulus is usually given simultaneously with the stimulator saying: "We are going to say /r/ (*r*at)."

Starting Position. Stimulator places fingers in position on respondent's face. As the manipulation is initiated: lips parted; mandible lowered slightly from position of closure; tongue in customary, relaxed position; vocal folds vibrating.

Simultaneous Stimulation. Stimulator places fingers in position on respondent's face. As the manipulation takes place, the respondent may observe the stimulator's face and/or hear an auditory stimulus.

EXTRAORAL MANIPULATION /r/ (*r*at)

1. Assume starting position.
2. Place thumb and middle finger on lower lip points 2.
3. Move mandible downward.
4. Place thumb and middle finger of other hand between upper lip points 3 and 4 and begin a series of short oscillating movements.
5. Phonate. (The stimulation may signal phonation by placing little finger against respondent's larynx.)

If the above manipulation is not sufficient, use the additional manipulation procedures.

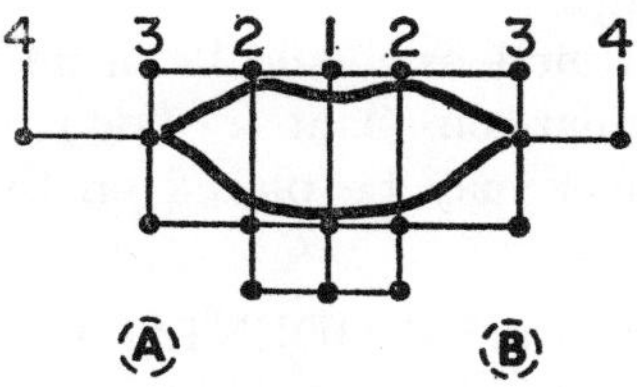

MANIPULATION MODEL: LIPS FORMAT.

ADDITIONAL MANIPULATION

1. Return to starting position.
2. Use thumb and middle finger of the other hand on mid-lip

points 3 to keep lips from assuming a rounded position as for /w/ (*w*e), which is a frequent substitution for the /r/ sound.
3. The sound of /ɑ/ (h*o*t) may be used as an initiating sound combined with quick oscillations used to stimulate /r/ (*r*at). The pressure applied by the thumb and middle finger at upper lip points 3 tends to bring the tongue up to the /r/ (*r*at) position.
4. The backs of the fingers of the lower hand may be used to press under the chin so that the tongue "humps up." (The pressure should be farther forward than that for the /ɝ/ (b*ir*d).
5. Phonate.

ALTERNATE MANIPULATION /r/ (*r*at)

1. Assume starting position.
2. Extend mandible.
3. Place thumb and middle finger on lower lip points 2.
4. Lower mandible slightly (remove fingers).
5. Press back of fingers of other hand under chin, farther forward than for /ɝ/ (b*ir*d), so that the tongue is pushed up against the maxillary alveolar ridge.
6. Phonate.

/r/ (*r*at) Response Analysis and Extraoral Cues

An /r/ is pronounced wherever it is found in the spelling by persons using general American speech. The /r/ in Southern, Eastern, and British is not always retroflex. The pronunciation may be a one-tap trill of *very,* a schwa of *sister,* or silent as in *far.* In these dialects, however, the initial /r/ of *rat,* the postconsonantal /r/ of *tree,* and the intervocalic /r/ of *very* are always pronounced in spite of allegation that they are the "r-less" dialects.

TONGUE. The one-tap trill used frequently between vowels in the East, England, and the South is made by one tap of the tongue tip against the alveolar ridge.

These allophonic distinctions should be of no concern to the stimulator. Strive for the regular consonant /r/ (*r*at).

VOCAL FOLDS. A finger may be placed on the respondent's larynx to signal phonation.

/r/ (*r*at) PHONODENTAL GUIDES

Chapter 5 gives details concerning preparation and placement of phonodental guides. Figures 5 and 6 in Chapter 5 illustrate the approximate points of lingual contact for the guides.

Phonodental guides and intraoral cues may be used independently or in combination with the extraoral manipulations. If intraoral stimulation is needed, one or more of the following phonodental guides may be utilized.

Denture Guides /r/ (*r*at)

Raise tongue sides: two denture guides placed in areas of Maxillary Second Bicuspids and First Molars (15-16 and 25-26).

Dental Floss Guides /r/ (*r*at)

Raise tongue sides: two knotted dental floss guides placed between Maxillary Second Bicuspids and First Molars (15-16 and 25-26). If placement is difficult, one stretched dental floss guide placed against crowns of Maxillary Second Bicuspids (15-25) or slightly posterior is suggested. These guides may be combined effectively with submandibular pressure.

Stemmed Wire Guides /r/ (*r*at)

Raise tongue tip and body: forked stemmed wire guide used to push tongue body and tip back and up slightly posterior to the Maxillary Second Bicuspids (15 and 25).

Cue Sticks /r/ (*r*at)

A tongue depressor may be used to elevate tongue body and tip.

/r/ (*r*at)* SELECTED PHONEME CHARACTERISTICS

DEVELOPMENTAL AGE:[1]

-r, -rk, -rm, -mr, -nr, -pr, -kr, -br, -dr, -gr = 3.5 yrs.; r-, -r-, pr-, tr-, kr-, br-, dr-, -rt, -fr = 4 yrs.; gr-, fr- = 4.5 yrs.; -rp, -rd, -rf, -rn, -shr, str-, -mbr = 5 yrs.; -rb, -rg, -rth, -thr, -str, -rst, -rj, -rch = 6 yrs.; thr-, shr-, skr-, spr-, -skr = 7 yrs.; -tr = 8 yrs.

FREQUENCY OF OCCURRENCE OF PHONEME:[2]

3.31%; ninth in occurrence

VISUAL INTELLIGIBILITY:[3]

50% to 90%; composite 62%

VISUAL CONFUSION:[4]

not given

AUDITORY INTELLIGIBILITY IN MILD-TO-SEVERE HEARING IMPAIRMENTS:[5]

58%

AUDITORY CONFUSION:[6]

/w, r, l/ (*w*e, *r*at, *l*et)

RELATIVE PHONETIC POWER:[7]

210 (range of 1 to 680)

---

* The symbol /r/ represents all allophones of the consonant /r/ in all positions of the word.

PHONEMIC CONFUSION:[8]
/r/ (*r*at), /w/ (*w*e),
/l/ (*l*et), /j/ (*y*et)
TYPICAL SPELLING:
r (*r*at); *rr* (ho*rr*id); *rh*(*rh*ododendron); *rrh* (cata*rrh*); *wr* (*wr*ite)

/r/ (*r*at) PRACTICE MATERIALS

The sound to be stimulated is /r/ (*r*at). Only those words and phrases in which the respondent can articulate all of the sounds correctly, except for the target phoneme, should be utilized for practice. The same stipulation applies to the practice materials provided at the end of this Section.

/r/ (*r*at)

/ɑ/ rock, rod, rotten, robin; /u/ roof, root, ruby, room; /i/ real, reed, Rita, reap; /ɑu/ round, rowdy, around, hour; /ɑi/ right, rye, rifle, riot; /ou/ road, rope, roll, rodeo; /ei/ ray, rail, rake, radio; /ɔ/ raw; /ɔi/ Roy, Royce; /ɪ/ rib, ring, rink, rear; /ɛ/ red, wren; /æ/ raft, rat, raffia, rattle; /ʊ/ cook, rook; /ʌ/ rut, rug, run, rub; /ə/ around. *Phrases:* A red wren ran around a robin. Roy and Rita are rowdy. Run, Ruby, run. Rats and raccoons are near the ravine.

Stimulation Unit 32

Phonetic Symbol and Representative Word: /j/ (*y*et)

Symbol Systems

International Phonetic Alphabet: /j/
Webster's New Collegiate Dictionary (1965): y
Thorndike-Barnhardt Comprehensive Dictionary (1951): y
Northampton Charts (Yale, 1946): y-

Topographical Relationships of Phoneme Production
/j/ (*y*et) voiced lingua-palatal fricative semivowel glide
MANDIBLE:
slightly lowered
LIPS:
neutral position
TONGUE:
Tip—at or near base of lower front teeth
Body—arched and forward
Sides—in contact with upper molars

[1-8] *Ibid.* (see p. 79).

AIRSTREAM:
forced through narrow opening between arched tongue and palate
NASAL PORT:
closed
VOCAL FOLDS:
vibrating

Stimulation Procedures

VISUAL-AUDITORY MODEL. A model demonstration is provided by the manipulation of the stimulator's face while the respondent observes. An auditory stimulus is usually given simultaneously as the stimulator is saying. "We are going to say /j/ (*y*et)."

STARTING POSITION. Respondent's articulators should be in the starting position before the manipulation is initiated: lips parted, mandible lowered slightly from positon of closure, tongue in customary, relaxed position, vocal folds not vibrating.

SIMULTANEOUS STIMULATION. Stimulator places fingers in position on respondent's face. As the manipulation takes place, the respondent may observe the stimulator's face and/or hear an auditory stimulus.

EXTRAORAL MANIPULATION /j/ (*y*et)

1. Assume starting position.
2. Place thumb and middle finger of one hand on upper lip points 2.
3. Place thumb and middle finger of other hand on lower lip points 2.
4. Press inward and slide fingers simultaneously *toward* mid-lip points 3.
5. Interrupt the sliding movement of lower hand before reaching mid-lip points 3.
6. Lower mandible sharply as a quick expulsion of air is produced.
7. Begin phonation and move immediately into position for succeeding sound. (The stimulator may signal phonation by placing little finger on respondent's larynx.)

If the above manipulation is not sufficient, use the additional manipulation.

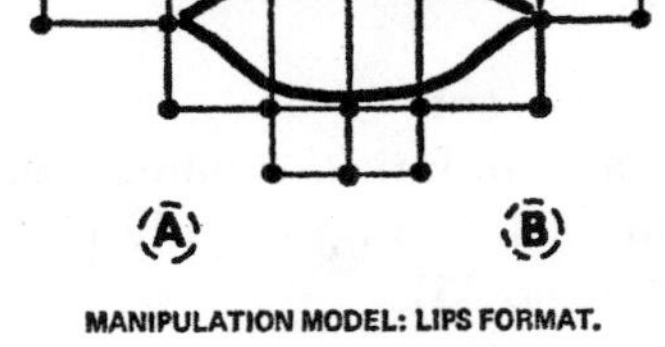

MANIPULATION MODEL: LIPS FORMAT.

ADDITIONAL MANIPULATION

The use of /ɑ/ (c*a*lm, l*o*t) following the stimulation for /j/ (*y*et) is helpful because it requires lowering of the mandible.

An /i/ (b*e*) sound may be used as a starting position for stimulating the /j/ (*y*et). With the sudden lowering of the mandible to /ɑ/ (c*a*lm, l*o*t) sound, the fricative quality of /j/ (*y*et) is usually achieved.

/j/ (*y*et) Response Analysis and Extraoral Cues

TONGUE. The tongue position for the /j/ (*y*et) is similar to that for the /i/ (*i*t).

ARTICULATORS. The articulators quickly assume the position of the vowel following /j/ (*y*et).

AIRSTREAM. The airstream gives a stronger exhalation as /j/ (*y*et) blends into the following vowel.

VOCAL FOLDS. A finger may be placed on the respondent's larynx to signal phonation.

/j/ (*y*et) PHONODENTAL GUIDES

Chapter 5 gives details concerning preparation and placement of phonodental guides. Figures 5 and 6 in Chapter 5 illustrate the approximate points of lingual contact for the guides.

Phonodental guides and intraoral cues may be used independently or in combination with the extraoral manipulations. If intraoral stimulation is needed, one or more of the following phonodental guides may be utilized.

Denture Guides /j/ (*y*et)

Raise tongue sides: two denture guides placed in areas of Maxillary Second Bicuspids and First Molars (15-16 and 25-26).

Dental Floss Guides /j/ (*y*et)

Raise tongue sides: two knotted dental floss guides placed between Maxillary Second Bicuspids and First Molars (15-16 and 25-26). If placement is difficult, one stretched dental floss guide placed against crowns of Maxillary Second Bicuspids (15-25) or slightly posterior is suggested. These guides may be combined effectively with submandibular pressure.

Stemmed Wire Guides /j/ (*y*et)

Raise tongue body and tip: forked stemmed wire guide used to push tongue body and tip back and up slightly posterior to the Maxillary Second Bicuspids (15 and 25).

Cue Sticks /j/ (*y*et)

A tongue depressor may be used to elevate tongue body and tip.

/j/ (*y*et) SELECTED PHONEME CHARACTERISTICS

DEVELOPMENTAL AGE:[1]

y-, -y-, = 3.5 yrs.

FREQUENCY OF OCCURRENCE OF PHONEME:[2]

2.40%; fifteenth in order of occurrence

VISUAL INTELLIGIBILITY:[3]

not given

VISUAL CONFUSION:[4]

/s, z, ʒ, t, dʒ, j/ (*s*o, *z*one, a*z*ure, *t*o, *j*am, *y*et)

AUDITORY INTELLIGIBILITY IN MILD-TO-SEVERE HEARING IMPAIRMENTS:[5]

41%

AUDITORY CONFUSION:[6]

/ʒ, z, v, ð, dʒ, j/ (a*z*ure, *z*one, *v*an, *th*is, *j*am, *y*et)

RELATIVE PHONETIC POWER:[7]

not given

PHONEMIC CONFUSION:[8]

/j/ (*y*et), /l/ (*l*et), /r/ (*r*at), /i/ (b*e*)

TYPICAL SPELLING:

y (*y*et); *i* (un*i*on); /j/ (hallelu*j*ah); *e* (*e*we); *u*(*u*nit)

/j/ (*y*et) PRACTICE MATERIALS

The sound to be stimulated is /j/ (*y*et). Only those words and phrases in which the respondent can articulate all of the sounds correctly, except the target phoneme, should be utilized for practice. The same stipulation applies to the practice materials provided at the end of this Section.

/j/ (*y*et)

/ɑ/ beyond, yacht; /u/ Matthew, you; /i/ ye, yeast; /ɑu/ yowl; /ɑi/ yipe; /iu/ feud, view, tube, duty; /ou/ yoke, Tokyo; /ei/ yea; /ɔ/ yaw, yawn; /ɔi/ buoyant; /ɪ/ year, Yiddish, yip, dominion; /ɛ/ yes, yet; /æ/ Yankee, yam, yap, yak; /ʌ/ young; /ə/ million, opinion. *Phrases:* The yacht cost a million. You and Matthew should marry this year. Don't give your opinion yet.

COMPARATIVE PRACTICE MATERIALS

SECTION I: FRICATIVES AND SEMIVOWELS

The sounds to be stimulated are /hw, w, l, r, and j/. Only those words and phrases in which the respondent can articulate all of the

[1-8] *Ibid.* (see p. 79).

sounds correctly, except the target phoneme, should be utilized for practice.

	/hw/ (*wh*at)	/w/ (*w*e)	/l/ (*l*et)	/r/ (*r*at)	/j/ (*y*et)
INITIAL POSITION:	what	watt	lot	rot	yacht
	whit	wit	lit	rit	
	whet	wet	let	Rhett	yet
	while	wile	Lyle	rile	
	Will		Lil	rill	
		weep	leap	reap	
	whip		lip	rip	yip
FINAL POSITION:			ill		
			all	are	
			"L"	air	

Chapter 7

SUGGESTED TEACHING ORDER FOR STIMULATION UNITS

THE ORDER OF THE SOUNDS in Chapter 7 progresses from those most easily stimulated to those for which the stimulations are less well defined. This organization lends itself to the training of clinicians, teachers, and others who are to become stimulators. The assumption is made that the persons in training do not have any defective speech sounds.

This teaching order is also useful with respondents who have many articulatory errors. If phonemes are taught according to the following suggested list, the respondent will not practice other sounds that are defective while he is correcting the articulation of the target phoneme.

The suggested sequence is helpful to respondents with little or no speech. By learning the phonemes in this order, the respondent will add only one new sound at a time. If one of the phonemes listed early in the sequence is particularly difficult for a respondent, the stimulator can go forward with the learning of additional phonemes, taking care not to use any practice materials incorporating the faulty phoneme until it has been learned or corrected.

Stimulations may consist of either the extraoral manipulations or the phonodental guides. In some instances, it may be necessary to use both.

In Chapter 6, the Stimulation Units are arranged according to traditional order. These Units include detailed information concerning extraoral manipulations and the placement of phonodental guides. The Unit numbers from Chapter 6 are included in the following practice materials.

A summary of the extraoral manipulations and placement of the phonodental guides is given in the Appendix.

Each stimulator should teach the Units in the order appropriate to the needs of the individual respondent.

Practice Group A includes the extreme vowels and their diphthongs, that are used in the learning of the consonant sounds. The vowels presented in Group A are the most easily stimulated. The consonants in this Group are presented in a sequence based, in most instances, on the place of articulation. In this way, it is possible to point up the *differences* as well as the *similarities* of these sounds.

Practice Group B utilizes the remaining vowels, diphthong, and /ŋ, ʒ/ (si*ng*, a*z*ure). These sounds are less easily stimulated. All of the consonants except /ŋ, ʒ/ (si*ng*, a*z*ure) will have been learned in Group A, consequently special attention can be devoted to the vowels and diphthong presented in Group B.

When teaching the /iu, ju/ (m*u*sic, *you*) it should be kept in mind that both the /iu, ju/ (m*u*sic, *you*) are acceptable. Time should not be spent in trying to differentiate between them. The semivowel glide /j/ (*y*et) is usually used in the initial position as in *y*es or *y*et; the /iu/ in m*u*sic, f*ew*. Certain spellings following /t, d, n/ may be pronounced as /iu/ or /u/ depending upon choice and ease of pronunciation, for example, *tune, dew,* and *new.*

In Group B, the /ɚ/ (sist*er*) is given only in the final position, since that is the position in which the phoneme is most often found.

SUGGESTED TEACHING ORDER FOR STIMULATION UNITS

GROUP A

Consonants	*Vowels and Diphthongs*						
	/ɑ/ #8 (calm, lot)	/i/ #1 (be)	/u/ #5 (boot)	/o, ou/ #13 (obey, go)	/ai/ #12 (mice)	/au/ #14 (cow)	/iu, ju/ #16 (music, *you*)
/h/ #23 (*h*at)	ah	"E"	"oo"	oh	eye	Ow!	you
	ha	he	who	ho	high	how	Hugh
	How high! Ho ho, ha ha, hee hee! Ah, Hugh!						
/p/ #20	Pa	pea	Pooh	Poe	pie	Pow	Pugh
	hop	heap	hoop	Hope			
	Pop	peep	poop	pope	pipe		
	You eye Pa. I owe you. Hi, Hope! Papa hop!						
/b/ #20 (*b*e)	bah	bee	boo	bow	buy	bow	
	bop	beep					
	Bow, Hugh. Buy pie. Hop, Papa.						
/m/ #17 (*m*e)	Ma	me	moo	Moe	my	Mau Mau	mew
	Mom						
	mop			mope			
	My hoop. By whom? You bomb. My Mom.						

Consonants	*Vowels and Diphthongs*						
	/ɑ/ #8 (c*a*lm, l*o*t)	/i/ #1 (b*e*)	/u/ #5 (b*oo*t)	/o, ou/ #13 (*o*bey, g*o*)	/ɑi/ #12 (m*i*ce)	/ɑu/ #14 (c*ow*)	/iu, ju/ #16 (m*u*sic, *you*)
/t/ #21		tea	two	toe	tie		
(*t*o)	tot		toot	tote	tight	tout	
	Tom	team	tomb	tome	time		
	hot	heat	hoot		height		
	pot	peat		Pote		pout	
	bought	beat	boot	boat	bite	bout	butte
	Mott	meat	moot	moat	might		mute
	Two bought tea. You type. I bought peat. Tom might buy meat.						
/d/ #21		"D"	do	dough	die	Dow	due
(*d*o)	Dodd	deed	dude	dodo	died	Dowd	
	Dom	deem	doom	dome	dime		
	Dot			dote		doubt	duty
	hod	heed	who'd	hoed	hide	howdy	dupe
		bead	booed	bode	bide	bowed	imbued
	mod	mead	mood	mode			mewed
	Tod	teed		toad	tied		
		deep	dupe	dope			
	Don't type. Do you date Todd? Don't doubt Dot.						

/n/ #18		knee	knew	know	nigh	now	new
(*no*)	non		noon	known	nine	noun	
	not	neat	Newt	note	night		Newt
	nod	need	nude	node			nude
	Don	dean	dune	Doan	dine	down	dune
	bonbon	bean	boon	bone			
		mean	moon	moan	mine		immune

He knew me. I need to know Dean. You dine at nine tonight.

/k/ #22		key	coup	Coe		cow	cue
(*keep*)	cock			coke			
	cop	keep	coop	cope			Cupid
	cot			coat			cute
	cod	keyed	cooed	code		cowed	cued
	con	keen	coon	cone			Kuhne
	pock	peak		poke	pike		puke
	bock	beak			bike		
	mock	meek		Moak	Mike		
	tock	teak	Tooke		tyke		
	dock	Deek	duke		dike		duke

Cook meat. Duke, cue Mike. Keep it, Katie.

Consonants	*Vowels and Diphthongs*						
	/ɑ/ #8 (*ca*lm, l*o*t)	/i/ #1 (b*e*)	/u/ #5 (b*oo*t)	/o, ou/ #13 (*o*bey, g*o*)	/ɑi/ #12 (m*i*ce)	/ɑu/ #14 (c*ow*)	/iu, ju/ #16 (m*u*sic, *you*)
/g/ #22 (*g*o)				go	guy		
	got			goat		gout	
	God			goad	guide		
	gone		goon			gown	
	dog	league					
	cog						

You cook goat meat. Guide Mike. Keep dog down.

Consonants	/ɑ/ #8 (*ca*lm, l*o*t)	/i/ #1 (b*e*)	/u/ #5 (b*oo*t)	/o, ou/ #13 (*o*bey, g*o*)	/ɑi/ #12 (m*i*ce)	/ɑu/ #14 (c*ow*)	/iu, ju/ #16 (m*u*sic, *you*)
/hw/ #29 (*wh*at)		whee		whoa	why?		whew
	what	wheat			white		

Why go to town now? My white gown. What wheat?

Consonants	/ɑ/ #8 (*ca*lm, l*o*t)	/i/ #1 (b*e*)	/u/ #5 (b*oo*t)	/o, ou/ #13 (*o*bey, g*o*)	/ɑi/ #12 (m*i*ce)	/ɑu/ #14 (c*ow*)	/iu, ju/ #16 (m*u*sic, *you*)
/w/ #29 (*w*e)		we	woo	woe	why!	wow	
	walk	week			wipe		
	wad	weed	wooed	woad	wide	wowed	
	wan	wean			wine		
	wok	weak		woke			

Why do you weep? He got weak wine.

/f/ #24	fa	fee	Fu		fie		few
(*f*ace)	fought	feet		foe	fight		
		feed	food				feud
	Few fight. Feed tom. Do not mock me. We fight; you weep.						
/v/ #24		"V"			vie	vow	view
(*v*an)		heave		hove	hive		
		peeve					
			move	mauve			
	Move on, Kuhne. He hove to. How white? I vow to fight!						
					thigh		
/θ/ #25			booth	both			
(*th*in)		teeth	tooth				
		Keith					
	Both teeth come out. Few fight Keith.						
/ð/ #25		thee		though	thy	thou	
(*th*is)		teethe			tithe		
	You tithe. I do not teethe now.						

Consonants	Vowels and Diphthongs						
	/ɑ/ #8 (*ca*lm, l*o*t)	/i/ #1 (b*e*)	/u/ #5 (b*oo*t)	/o, ou/ #13 (*o*bey, g*o*)	/ɑi/ #12 (m*i*ce)	/ɑu/ #14 (c*ow*)	/iu, ju/ #16 (m*u*sic, *you*)
/s/ #26 (*s*o)		see	sue	so	sigh	sow	
	sop	seap	soup	soap			
	sot	seat	suit		sight		
	sod	seed	sued	sewed	sighted	Saudi	
	San	seen	soon	sown	sign		
	sock	seek		soak			
		cease	Seuss			souse	
	moss		moose		mice	mouse	
		niece	noose		nice		
		geese	goose				

Did Sue see it? The goose can be cooked. The mouse went outside.

/z/ #26 (*z*one)			zoos	Zoe			
		he's	whose	hoze	highs	house	hues
	Pa's	peas		pose	pies		pews
		bees	boos	bows	buys	bows	abuse
	Ma's		moos	mows			mews
		tease	two's	toes	ties		
		knees	news	nose			news
		keys	coos			cows	cues
		fees					fuse
	vase	"V's"			vies	vows	views
		"Z's"	zoos				

The vase was a white piece. His niece's name is not in the news. The man moved out of that zone.

/ʃ/ #27	Shah	she	shoe	show	shy		
(*sh*oe)	shop	sheep					
	shot	sheet	shoot	shoat		shout	
	shod	she'd	shoed	showed	shied		
		sheen		shown	shine		
	shock	sheik					

She washed the sheets. The moon shone. They shut the sheep in the pens.

/tʃ/ #28	cha cha		choo choo			chow	
(*ch*in)	chop	cheap					
			chewed		chide		chewed
	chock	cheek		choke			
		peach	pooch	poach		pouch	
	botch	beach					

Cheap meat is tough. The peach punch was too sweet.

/dʒ/ #28		gee	Jew	Joe	Jai		Jew
(*j*am)	job		Jube	Jobe	gibe		
	Jock		Juke	joke			
	John	Jean	June	Joan			June
	jog						
	jaws		Jews	Joe's	Jai's		Jews

The joke is on June. Jim beached the boat. A jig is much fun to dance.

Consonants	*Vowels and Diphthongs*						
	/ɑ/ #8 (calm, lot)	/i/ #1 (be)	/u/ #5 (boot)	/o, ou/ #13 (obey, go)	/ɑi/ #12 (mice)	/ɑu/ #14 (cow)	/iu, ju/ #16 (music, *you*)
/l/ #30 (*l*et)	la	lea	Lu	low	lie		
	lop	leap	loop	lope			
	lob		lube	lobe			
			loom	loam	line		
	lot		loot		light	lout	
		lead	lewd	load	lied	loud	
	Lon	lean	loon	loan	line		
	lock	leak	Luke	Logue			
	log	league					
		leaf		loaf	life		
		leave			live		
	loss	lease	loose		lice	louse	
		Lee's	lose	lows	lies		
		peal	pool	pole	pile	Powell	
		beal	buhl	bowl	bile	bowel	Beull
	moll	meal		mole	mile		mule
		teal	tool	toll	tile	towel	
	doll	deal	duel	dole	dial	dowel	duel
		kneel	Newell	knoll	nile		renewal
		keel	cool	coal	Kyle	cowle	
		feel	fool	foal	file	fowl	feud
		veal			vile		
	Sol	seal		soul			

Joe likes to listen to the large juke box. Don't lean on the fence. Leave the whole load.

/r/ #31	rah	re	rue	row	rye	row	
(*r*at)		reap		rope	ripe		
	rob			robe			
		ream	room	Rome	rhyme		
	rot		root	rote	write	rout	
	rod	reed	rude	road	ride		
	Ron		rune	roan	Rhine		
	rock	reek					
		reef	roof		rife		
		wreath	Ruth				
					writhe		
	Ross	Reece	ruse		rice	Rouse	
	car	reel	rule	role	rile		
				core			
					fire		
			lure		sire	sour	

All roads lead to Rome. Can you row up the Rhine? The bush had many red roses.

/j/ #32	yah	ye			you
(*y*et)			yoke		uke

You showed me the yellow robe. You put the yoke on the oxen.

GROUP B

Consonants	*Vowels and Diphthongs*									
	/e, ei/ #12 (*va*cation, g*a*te)	/ɪ/ #2 (*i*t)	/ɛ/ #3 (b*e*t)	/æ/ #4 (*a*t)	/ʊ/ #6 (f*oo*t)	/ɔ/ #7 (s*aw*, w*a*r)	/ɔi/ #15 (b*oy*)	/ʌ/ #9 (c*u*p)	/ɝ/ #16 (b*ir*d)	/ɚ/ #16 (sist*er*)
/h/ #23 (*h*at)	hay					haw	hoi	hub	her	
		hip	hep	hap	hoop					
							Hoyt	hut	hurt	
		hid	head	had	hood	hawed		Hud	heard	harder
		hick	heck	hack	hook	hawk		Huck		
	Hague			hag		hog		hug		
		him	hem	ham				Hun	Herm	hammer
	haze	his		has		Hawes			hers	
				hash				hush	Hirsch	
	hail	hill	hell	Hal		haul	Hoyle	hull	hurl	
		hear	hair							

Have you had hash? Hal has hurt his hand. Herm hid his loop. I heard you had her hat.

/p/ #20	pay					paw	poi		purr	
(*p*at)	Pape	pip	pep	pap				pup		
	pate	pit	pet	pat	put			putt	pert	putter
	paid		ped	pad		pawed		Pud		
	pain	pin	pen	pan		pawn		pun		
		pick	peck	pack				Puck	perk	pucker
	pale	pill	pell	pal	pull	pall			Pearl	
		peer	pear		poor				purr	
	tape	tip		tap						
	nape	nip		nap						
	shape	ship	Shep							
	rape	rip	rep	rap				Rupp		wrapper

Pam picked up the puppy. Peg pawned the pearl. Wrap the pen. Put the pig in his pen.

/b/ #20	bay			baa			boy		burr	
(*b*e)	babe	bib								
	bait	bit	bet	bat		bought		but	Bert	batter
		bid	bed	bad			Boyd	bud	bird	bidder
	bane	bin	Ben	ban				bun	burn	burner
	bake	Bic	beck	back	book	balk		buck	Burke	backer
		big	beg	bag		bog		bug	Berg	Berger
	base		Bess	bass		boss	Boyce	bus	burse	baser
	bale	bill	bell		bull	ball	boil		Burl	boiler
				cab				cub	curb	

Bat bought a baby bib. Bert bagged a bird. A cub bit a boy. Bake a ham.

Consonants	*Vowels and Diphthongs*									
	/e, ei/ #12 (v*a*cation, g*a*te)	/ɪ/ #2 (*i*t)	/ɛ/ #3 (b*e*t)	/æ/ #4 (*a*t)	/ʊ/ #6 (f*oo*t)	/ɔ/ #7 (s*aw*, w*a*r)	/ɔi/ #15 (b*oy*)	/ʌ/ #9 (c*u*p)	/ɝ/ #16 (b*ir*d)	/ɚ/ #16 (sist*er*)
/m/ #17	may					maw			Myrrh	Mayor
(*m*e)	mate	mitt	met	mat				mutt	Myrt	matter
	made	mid		mad		Maude		mud		murder
	Mame	Min	men	man						manner
	make	Mick		Mac		mock		muck	Merck	maker
	tame	Tim		tam		Tom		tum	term	tamer
	dame	dim		dam				dumb		dumber
	came	Kim	Kem					come		
	same	Sim		Sam				some	sermon	
	James	Jim	gem	jam					germ	
	lame	limb	Lem	lamb						lamer
		rim	Rehm	ram				rum		

May met Tim and Bert. Men might tame a bear. Some seem happy. Come home Monday.

/t/ #21	take	tick		tack	took			tuck	Turk	Tucker
(*to*)		tin	ten	tan				ton	turn	Turner
	tale	till	tell			tall	toil			toiler
		tear	tear		tour					
	date		debt						dirt	
	Nate	knit	net	knat		nought		nut		
	Kate	kit		cat		caught		cut	Curt	cutter
	gate		get	gat				gut	Gert	gutter
	wait	wit	wet							wetter
	fate	fit		fat	foot	fought				fitter
		sit	set	sat	soot	sought			cert	setter
	late	lit	let							later
	rate	writ	Rhett	rat	root	wrought		rut		

Take a turn. Kate may knit a cap. He tore a page in two. A cat caught a bird.

/d/ #21		did	dead	dad				dud		daughter
(*do*)	Dake	Dick	deck					duck	Dirk	dicker
	deign	din	den	Dan		dawn		dun		dinner
	Dale	dill	dell				Doyle	dull		duller
		dear	dare							
		kid	Ked	cad	could	cawed		cud	curd	
	fade		fed	fad						
		Sid	said	sad		sawed			surd	solder
	shade		shed	shad	should					
	laid	lid	lead	lad		laud	Lloyd			larder
	raid	rid	read							raider

Duke ate duck at dinner. Sid bought a ticket. She fed seed to the birds. Can you decorate the hall?

Consonants						*Vowels and Diphthongs*				
	/e, ei/ #12 (*va*cation, g*a*te)	/ɪ/ #2 (*i*t)	/ɛ/ #3 (b*e*t)	/æ/ #4 (*a*t)	/ʊ/ #6 (f*oo*t)	/ɔ/ #7 (s*aw*, w*a*r)	/ɔi/ #15 (b*oy*)	/ʌ/ #9 (c*u*p)	/ɝ/ #16 (b*ir*d)	/ɚ/ #16 (sist*er*)
/n/ #18		nick	neck	knack	nook					
(*n*o)	nail	nil	Nell					null		
		near				nor				nearer
	cane	kin	ken	can			coin		Kearn	canner
	Wayne	win	wen					won		Werner
	feign	fin	fen	fan		fawn		fun	fern	
	vain			van		Vaughn			Vern	vainer
	thane	thin								
			then	than						
	sane	sin						sun		saner
	Shayne	shin				Sean		shun		
	chain	chin		Chan					churn	
	Jane	gin		Jan			join			
	lane	Lynn				lawn	loin		learn	learner
	rain		wren	ran				run		runner

Nell hurt her shin. Wayne may win. Neither Shayne nor Lynn can bake. Mother gave Nan some money.

/k/ #22	cake	kick			cook	caulk			Kirk	cooker
(*k*eep)	cave			calve					curve	cover
	case	kiss		Cass				cuss	curse	kisser
	kale	kill		Cal		call	coil	cull	curl	curler
				care	Coor				cur	
	sake	sick		sack				suck		sicker
	shake	Schick		shack	shook			shuck	shirk	shaker
	lake	lick		lack	look			luck	lurk	liquor
	rake	Rick	wreck	wrack	rook					wrecker

Do you like chocolate cake? Tell Cal to take a rake. Call Kirk about Mike's cake.

/g/ #22	gave	give								giver
(*g*o)	Gayle	Gil		gal		gall		gull	girl	

Gill gave the girl a dog. Gayle came to rake the lawn. Look for the cave by the lake.

/ŋ/ #23		sing		sang		song		sung		
(si*ng*)		ping		pang						
		Bing		bang		bong				
		Ming								
				Tang		tong		tongue		
						long		lung		

Bing paid me. Ping pong can be tame. A tongue ought to be pink.

Consonants — *Vowels and Diphthongs*

	/e, ei/ #12 (v*a*cation, g*a*te)	/ɪ/ #2 (*i*t)	/ɛ/ #3 (b*e*t)	/æ/ #4 (*a*t)	/ʊ/ #6 (f*oo*t)	/ɔ/ #7 (s*aw*, w*a*r)	/ɔi/ #15 (b*oy*)	/ʌ/ #9 (c*u*p)	/ɝ/ #16 (b*ir*d)	/ɚ/ #16 (sist*er*)
/hw/ #29	whey								whir	
(*wh*at)		whip								
		whim		wham						
				whack						

Ben ate whey. He may make money on a whim.

/w/ #29	weigh					Waugh			were	
(*w*e)			web							weber
									worm	
	wait	wit	wet							waiter
	wade		wed		would				word	
	wane	win	wen					won		Werner
	wake	wick		WAC		WOC			work	worker
		wing				wong				
	wail	will	well		wool	wall				

Weigh each word. A tail wagging dog does not bite. Would a waiter work with Wayne?

/f/ #24	phase	fizz	fez					fuzz	furs	offers
(*f*ace)	fail	fill	fell		full	fall	foil		furl	
		fear		fare		for				wayfarer
		riff		raff	roof			rough		rougher

He fell off a roof. He hit his face in a fight. Unfurl the flag on a holiday.

/v/ #24	veil			Val			voile			
(*v*an)	save	sieve		salve					serve	savor
	shave							shove		shaver
	lave	live						love		

A sailor likes to live on a ship. Val saved the wayfarer. The veil was of voile.

/θ/ #25				hath					
(*th*in)		pith		path					Perth
			Beth	bath					birth
		myth		math		moth			mirth
			death					doth	dirth
	faith								furth

Beth may miss math. The wing of the moth was tan and white.

/ð/ #25	bathe
(*th*is)	lathe

The lathe was new. Bathe this boy. The thin man had faith.

Consonants	/e, ei/ #12 (*va*cation, g*a*te)	/ɪ/ #2 (*i*t)	/ɛ/ #3 (b*e*t)	/æ/ #4 (*a*t)	/ʊ/ #6 (f*oo*t)	/ɔ/ #7 (s*aw*, w*a*r)	/ɔi/ #15 (b*oy*)	/ʌ/ #9 (c*u*p)	/ɝ/ #16 (b*ir*d)	/ɚ/ #16 (sist*er*)
/s/ #26		sis		sass		sauce				pacer
(*s*o)	chase		chess				choice			
	lace		less	lass		loss				

Save some ice cream for me. Sam's choice is difficult. The policeman took care of that car.

Consonants	/e, ei/ #12	/ɪ/ #2	/ɛ/ #3	/æ/ #4	/ʊ/ #6	/ɔ/ #7	/ɔi/ #15	/ʌ/ #9	/ɝ/ #16	/ɚ/ #16
/z/ #26	zane		zen							
(*z*one)				Zac	zook					
		zig		zag						
		zing								
	pays					pause	poise			
	bays						boys	buzz	burns	
	maze									
	daze							does		
						gnaws	noise			
	faze	fizz	fez					fuzz	furs	
	jays			jazz		jaws	joys			
	lays	Liz				laws				
	raise			razz			Roy's			

Zac is Roy's lawyer. Liz finds joy in jazz.

/ʃ/ #27	shape	ship								
(*sh*oe)	shame			sham						
	shade		shed	shad						
	Shane	shin				Sean		shun		
	shake	Schick		shack	shook			shuck	shirk	shirker
	shale	schill	sheel	shall		shawl			Shurl	
		sheer		share						

The shoe is the wrong shape. Shurl should shun the shirker.

/ʒ/ #27	beige	
(a*z*ure)		

The beige shawl is sheer. Shall I shake the moth off the bush? Sean looks at the azure sky.

/tʃ/ #28	chain	chin		Chan					churn	
(*ch*in)		chick	check					Chuck		
	chafe			chaff						
		cheer		chair						
		pitch		patch					perch	
		Mitch		match				much		
		witch								
		rich	wretch							

Mitch had a patch on his chin. Watch the witch. The chair matched the window shade.

/dʒ/ #28	jays			jazz		jaws	joys			merger
(*j*am)	jail	Jill	jell							
	rage	ridge	Reg							

Do blue jays eat bugs? Jazz has become the rage in music. *Jaws* is a famous motion picture.

Consonants	*Vowels and Diphthongs*									
	/e, ei/ #12 (v*a*cation, g*a*te)	/ɪ/ #2 (*i*t)	/ɛ/ #3 (b*e*t)	/æ/ #4 (*a*t)	/ʊ/ #6 (f*oo*t)	/ɔ/ #7 (s*aw*, w*a*r)	/ɔi/ #15 (b*oy*)	/ʌ/ #9 (c*u*p)	/ɝ/ #16 (b*ir*d)	/ɚ/ #16 (sist*er*)
/l/ #30		Lil						lull		curler
(*l*et)	layer	leer			lure					
	rail	rill					roil			

The layer cake is vanilla. Lil put a large curler in her hair. Jack and Jill fell down the hill.

/r/ #31	rate	Rit	Rhett	rat		wrought	Roy	rut		rupture
(*r*at)		near	rare	rare	Ruhr	roar				bearer

A rare jewel is of great value. He came near to the edge of the road. Riding a horse can be dangerous.

/j/ #32			yes							
(*y*et)			yet							
	yea		yeah			yaw				lawyer

Yes, the youngster will join the yacht club. Yesterday, you met Yvonne.

SECTION IV
Appendices

SUMMARY OF EXTRAORAL AND INTRAORAL STIMULATIONS

Phonemes and Unit Numbers	*Extraoral Manipulations*	*Phonodental Guides and FDI* Numbers*
/i/ (b*e*) #1	Place thumb and middle finger on upper lip points 2; slide toward upper lip points 3; phonate.	One floss guide between Mandibular Central Incisors (31-41); or shorter stem to position tongue tip behind Mandibular Central Incisors (31-41); or two guides between Maxillary Second Bicuspids and First Molars (15-16 and 25-26); or tips of forked guide in area of Maxillary Second Bicuspids and First Molars (15-16 and 25-26).
/ɪ/ (*i*t) #2	Place side of index finger on lower lip point 1 and draw line between lower lip points 1 and mid-chin point 1; phonate.	Same as above.
/e/ (v*a*cation) #12 Element of /ei/ (g*a*te)	Place thumb and middle finger on mid-chin points 2; press; phonate.	One floss guide between Mandibular Central Incisors (31-41); or shorter stem to position tongue tip behind

* Federation Dentaire Internationale Tooth Numbering System.

Phonemes and Unit Numbers	*Extraoral Manipulations*	*Phonodental Guides and FDI* Numbers*
		Mandibular Central Incisors (31-41); or two guides between Mandibular Central Incisors and Lateral Incisors (31-32 and 41-42); or two guides or tips of forked stemmed guides between Maxillary Second Bicuspids and First Molars (15-16 and 25-26).
/ɛ/ (b*e*t) #3	Press tip of index finger on lower lip point 1; phonate.	One floss guide between Mandibular Central Incisors (31-41); or shorter stem to position tongue tip behind Mandibular Central Incisors (31-41); or two guides or tips of forked stemmed wire guide between Maxillary Second Bicuspids and First Molars (15-16 and 25-26).
/æ/ (*a*t) #4	Place thumb and middle finger on lower lip points 2; press; move half-way to mid-lip points 3; phonate.	One floss guide between Mandibular Central Incisors (31-41); or shorter stem to position tongue tip behind Mandibular Central Incisors (31-41); or two guides between Mandibular Cuspids and First Bicuspids (33-34 and 43-44); or stemmed reflexor used to produce low tongue position.

Phonemes and Unit Numbers	*Extraoral Manipulations*	*Phonodental Guides and FDI* Numbers*
/u/ (b*oo*t) #5	Place thumb and middle finger on mid-lip points 3; direct corners of mouth toward mid-lip line 1; phonate.	Two denture or floss guides; or tips of forked stemmed guide between Maxillary First Molars and Second Molars (16-17 and 26-27).
/ʊ/ (f*oo*t) #6	Place thumb and middle finger just above mid-lip points 3; place thumb and middle finger of other hand just below mid-lip points 3; bring lips into rounded, protruded position; phonate.	Same as above.
/o/ (*o*bey) #13 Element of /ou/ (g*o*)	Place thumb and middle finger on mid-lip points 3; direct corners of lips toward mid-line 1, forming rounded opening; phonate.	Same as /u, ʊ/ (b*oo*t, f*oo*t)
/ɔ/ (s*aw*, w*a*r) #7	Place thumb and middle finger on mid-lip points 3; place thumb and middle finger of other hand on lower lip points 2; shape lips into slightly oval form; phonate.	Stemmed reflexor used to stimulate low tongue position.
/ɑ/ (c*a*lm, l*o*t) #8	Place thumb and middle finger on mid-chin points 2; press inward and guide mandible downward; phonate.	Same as above.
/ʌ, ə/ (c*u*p, sof*a*) #9	Place thumb and middle finger on mid-chin points 2; relax tongue and lips; phonate.	Stemmed reflexor used to stimulate low tongue positions.

Phonemes and Unit Numbers	*Extraoral Manipulations*	*Phonodental Guides and FDI* Numbers*
/ɜ˞, ɚ/ (b*ir*d, sist*er*) #10	Place thumb and middle finger on mid-chin points 2; place same fingers of other hand on upper lip points 3; phonate.	Denture guides placed in area of Maxillary First Molars (16 and 26); or one stretched dental floss guide against crowns of Maxillary First Molars (16 and 26); or two knotted dental floss guides between Maxillary First and Second Molars (16-17 and 26-27); or forked stemmed wire guide used to push tongue body and tip back and up into area of Maxillary First Molars (16 and 26).
/ɑi/ (m*i*ce) #11	Place thumb and middle finger of one hand on lower lip points 2; phonate; press inward and slide fingers into "smile position."	See Units 8 and 1 for further details.
/ei/ (g*a*te) #12	Place thumb and middle finger on mid-chin 2; phonate; press inward and slide fingers into "smile position."	See Units 12 and 1 for further details or descriptions given elsewhere in this *Summary*.
/ou/ (g*o*) #13	Place thumb and middle finger on mid-lip points 3; direct corners of mouth toward mid-lip line 1; phonate; direct corners farther toward mid-lip line 1.	See Units 13 and 1 for further details or descriptions given earlier in this *Summary*.
/ɑu/ (c*ow*) #14	Place thumb and middle finger on mid-chin points	See Units 8 and 5 for further details or descrip-

Phonemes and Unit Numbers	*Extraoral Manipulations*	*Phonodental Guides and FDI* Numbers*
	2; phonate; direct corners of mouth toward mid-lip line 1.	tions given earlier in this *Summary.*
/ɔi/ (b*oy*) #15	Place thumb and middle finger on mid-lip points 3; place thumb and middle finger of other hand on lower lip points 2; shape lips into oval; phonate; press inward and slide fingers of lower hand toward mid-lip point 3, into "smile" position.	See Units 7 and 1 for further details or descriptions given earlier in this *Summary.*
/iu, ju/ (m*u*sic, *you*) #16	Place thumb and middle finger on lower lip points 2; slide toward mid-lip points 3; phonate; place thumb and middle finger of other hand on upper lip points 3; direct both hands towards mid-lip line 1.	See Units 1, 5 and 32 for details.
/m/ (*m*e) #17	Place thumb and middle finger on lower lip points 2; move lower lip toward mid-lip line; phonate.	None
/n/ (*n*o) #18	Place side of third finger along upper lip line between points 2; phonate.	One denture, floss, or longer stem guide in area of Maxillary Central Incisors (11-21).
/ŋ/ (si*ng*) #19	Place thumb and middle finger on submandibular points 3; press upward and inward firmly but gently; phonate.	Two floss guides between Maxillary First Molars and Second Molars (16-17 and 26-27); or a stretched floss guide

Phonemes and Unit Numbers	*Extraoral Manipulations*	*Phonodental Guides and FDI* Numbers*
		across Maxillary Second Molars (17 and 27); or single long stemmed guide touching area of lingua-velar contact.
/p, b/ (*p*at, *b*e) #20	Place thumb and middle finger on lower lip points 2; for /b/ (*b*e), add thumb and middle finger of other hand on upper lip points 2 and press lips together; phonate for /b/ (*b*e).	None
/t, d/ (*t*o, *d*o) #21	Place index finger on upper lip point 1; exert pressure; remove with flicking motion for /t/ (*t*o); phonate for /d/ (*d*o).	One denture, floss, or longer stem guide placed in area of Maxillary Central Incisors (11-21).
/k, g/ (*k*eep, *g*o) #22	Place thumb and middle finger on submandibular points 3; press upward and inward; release; phonate for /g/ (*g*o).	Two floss guides between Maxillary First Molars and Second Molars (16-17 and 26-27); or stretched floss guide across Maxillary Second Molars (17 and 27); or long stemmed guide touching place of lingua-velar contact.
/h/ (*h*at) #23	Lower Mandible; use hand to press inward and upward with sudden movement; just below the sternum; direct air stream through oral cavity.	None
/f, v/ (*f*ace, *v*an) #24	Place thumb and middle finger on lower lip line points 2; move lower lip	None

Phonemes and Unit Numbers	*Extraoral Manipulations*	*Phonodental Guides and FDI* Numbers*
	upward into approximation with edge of upper incisors; insert air stream; phonate for /v/ (*v*an).	
/θ, ð/ (*th*in, *th*is) #25	Lower Mandible; press index finger of each hand along upper lip and lower lip line points 3; air stream directed through lingua-alveolar opening; phonate for /ð/ (*th*is).	None
/s, z/ (*s*o, *z*one) #26	Place thumb and third finger on upper lip points 2; direct lips slightly toward upper lip points 3; emit air-stream through lingua-alveolar aperture; phonate for /z/ (*z*one).	Two floss guides between Maxillary Lateral Incisors and Cuspids (12-13 and 22-23) or between Mandibular Central Incisors and Lateral Incisors (31-32 and 41-42); or longer stem of double-ended guide for maxillary position or shorter stem for mandibular position.
/ʃ, ʒ/ (*sh*oe, a*z*ure) #27	Press thumb and third finger on lip points 3; press thumb and finger of other hand on lower lip points 3; move all fingers slightly toward mid-lip line; emit air-stream through lingua-alveolar aperture; phonate for /ʒ/ (a*z*ure).	Two denture or floss guides, or tips of forked guide between Maxillary Second Bicuspids and First Molars (15-16 and 25-26); or single long stemmed guide.
/tʃ, dʒ/ (*ch*in, *j*am) #28	Place second finger on upper lip point 1; press; remove with flicking	Two floss guides or tips of forked guide placed at Maxillary Cuspids and

Phonemes and Unit Numbers	*Extraoral Manipulations*	*Phonodental Guides and FDI* Numbers*
	motion; quickly press lower lip points 3; lower mandible sharply, followed by expulsion of air and air friction emitted through lingua-alveolar aperture; phonate for /dʒ/ (*j*am).	Bicuspids (13-14 and 23-24); or long stemmed guide.
/hw, w/ (*wh*at, *w*e) #29	Place thumb and third finger on mid-points 3; move lips into rounded position; for /hw/ (*wh*at) press inward and upward suddenly below sternum; phonate for /w/ (*w*e).	None
/l/ (*l*et) #30	Place thumb and third finger between upper lip points 2-3; press; phonate.	Three floss guides between Maxillary Central Incisors (11-21) and Cuspids and First Bicuspids (13-14 and 23-24); or tips of forked guide in area ofMaxillary Cuspids and Bicuspids (13-14 and 23-24); or single long stemmed guide to raise tongue and indicate contact areas.
/r/ (*r*at) #31	Place thumb and middle finger between upper lip points 3 and 4; use finger oscillation; phonate.	Two denture guides or two floss guides in areas of Maxillary Second Bicuspids and First Molars (15-16 and 25-26); or stretched floss guide against crown of Maxillary Second Bicuspids (15-25); or

Phonemes and Unit Numbers	*Phonodental Guides and*	*Extraoral Manipulations FDI* Numbers*
		forked guide used to push tongue body and tip back and up to or posterior to Maxillary Second Bicuspids (15-25).
/j/ (*y*et) #32	Place thumbs and middle fingers on upper and lower lip points 2; slide toward mid-lip points 3; interrupt sliding motion of lower hand and lower mandible sharply; phonate; immediately move into position for following phoneme.	Two denture or floss guides between Maxillary Second Bicuspids and First Molars (15-16 and 25-26) or stretched floss guide against crown of Maxillary Second Bicuspids (15-25); or forked guide used to push tongue body and tip back and up slightly posterior to Maxillary Second Bicuspids (15-25).

REFERENCES

Abbs, J. H.: The influence of the gamma motor system on jaw movements during speech: A theoretical framework and some preliminary observations. *J Speech Hear Res, 16:*175-200, 1973.

Abbs, J. H., Folkins, J. W., and Sivarajan, M.: Motor impairment following blockade of the infraorbital nerve: Implications for the use of anesthetization techniques in speech research. *J Speech Hear Res, 19:*19-35, 1976.

Akin, Johnnye: *And So We Speak.* Englewood Cliffs, P-H, 1958, pp. 10, 85.

Arndt, W. B., Gauer, J., Shelton, R. L., Crary, D., and Chisum, L.: Refinement of a test of oral stereognosis. In Bosma, J. F. (Ed.): *Second Symposium on Oral Sensation and Perception.* Springfield, Thomas, 1970, pp. 363-377.

ASHA, Necrology, Edna Hill Young. *10:*299, 1968.

ASHA, Necrology, Sara Stinchfield Hawk. *20:*23, 1978.

Baumell, J. J.: Trigeminal-facial nerve communications. *Arch Otolaryngol, 99:*34-44, 1974.

Berry, Mildred F.: *Language Disorders of Children: The Bases and Diagnoses.* New York, Appleton-Century-Crofts, Meredith Corp, 1969.

Borden, Gloria, Harris, Katherine, and Catena, L.: Oral feedback II. An electromyographic study of speech under nerve-block anesthesia. *J Phonetics, 1:*297-308, 1973.

Bosma, J. F. (Ed.): *Symposium on Oral Sensation and Perception.* Springfield, Thomas, 1967.

Bosma, J. F. (Ed.): *Second Symposium on Oral Sensation and Perception.* Springfield, Thomas, 1970.

Bosma, J. F. (Ed.): *Third Symposium on Oral Sensation and Perception, The Mouth of the Infant.* Springfield, Thomas, 1972.

Bowman, J. P.: *The Muscle Spindle and Neural Control of the Tongue.* Springfield, Thomas, 1971.

Breckwoldt, G. H.: The use of the artificial palate. *Volta Review, 50:*301-303, 1948.

Brutten, E. J., and Shoemaker, D. J.: *The Modification of Stuttering.* Englewood Cliffs, P-H, 1967, p. 7.

Cable, A. W.: Dynamic factors in moto-kinaesthetic method of speech correction. *Q J Speech, 31,* 1945.

Carhart, R.: Conservation of speech. In Davis, H.: *Hearing and Deafness.* New York, H, R, & W, 1960, pp. 388-393.

Carrell, J. A.: *Disorders of Articulation.* Englewood Cliffs P-H, 1968, p. 9.

Chalfant, J. C., and Scheffelin, Margaret A.: *Central Processing Dysfunctions in Children. NINDS Monograph No. 9.* Bethesda, National Institute of Neurological Diseases and Stroke, Public Health Service, National Institutes of Health, U. S. Department of Health, Education, and Welfare, 1969.

Chase, R. A.: Abnormalities in motor control secondary to congenital sensory deficits. In Bosma, J. F. (Ed.): *Symposium on Oral Sensation and Perception.* Springfield, Thomas, 1967, pp. 302-309.

Clark, Ruth M.: Speech pathology (logopedics) in the U.S.S.R. *ASHA*, 3, 1961.

Clark, Ruth M.: Application of the moto-kinesthetic method in the speech clinic. *South Speech J, 27*, 1962.

Clark, Ruth M.: The self concept of laryngectomees as shown by the W-A-Y test. *De Therapia Vocis et Laquelae*, Paris, 1968.

Clark, Ruth M., and Fitzpatrick, J. A.: Self concept in diagnosis and therapy. In Barbara, D. A. (Ed.): *The Psychotherapy of Stuttering.* Springfield, Thomas, 1962.

Clark, Ruth M., and Van Tine, Ruth: *Directions for Stimulating Speech by the Moto-Kinesthetic Method*, 1947. (This manual was mimeographed at the University of Denver, Speech Clinic.)

Class, L. W.: *Comparative Study of Normal Speakers and Speech Defectives with Regard to the Tactual-Kinesthetic Perception of Form with the Tongue.* Master's thesis, Ohio State University, 1956.

Cooper, S.: Muscle spindles in the intrinsic muscles of the human tongue. *J Physiol, 122:*193-202, 1953.

Cornett, R. O.: Cued speech. *Am Ann Deaf, 112:*3-13, 1967.

Critchley, M.: Disorders of corporeal awareness in parietal disease. In Wapner, S. and Werner, H. (Eds.): *The Body Concept.* New York, Random, 1965, p. 68.

Daniels, L. M., Sim, Joseph M., and Simon, J. F., Jr.: Plastics in pedodontics. *Dental Clinics of North America*, 1966.

Darley, F. L., Aronson, A. E., and Brown, J. R.: *Motor Speech Disorders.* Philadelphia, Saunders, 1975.

Denes, P. B., and Pinson, E. W.: *The Speech Chain.* Garden City, N. Y. Doubleday, 1966.

Dillydot: 1976 (Announcement gave address as: 171 Meadowbrook Road, Englewood, N. J. 07631.)

Dittman, Helen M.: *The Role of Proprioceptive Sensibilities in Speech Production.* Unpublished doctoral thesis, University of Denver, 1955, p. 132.

Dorland's Illustrated Medical Dictionary. Philadelphia, Saunders, 1965, pp. 872-3.

Dorn, J. A.: *Phonetic Context Analysis of General American Consonants and Vowels.* Unpublished master's thesis. Eastern Illinois University, 1974.

Eagleson, H. M.: A specially adapted mobile standing device (surfboard) for spinal cord injury patients. *Proceedings of Fifteenth Annual Clinical Spinal Cord Injury Conference,* Veterans Administration Hospital, West Roxbury, MA, 1966.

Eagleson, H. M.: Conversation with authors, 1972.

Eggermont, J. P.: Acquisition of language in a group of deaf children. *J Speech Hear Res, 3:*242-248, 1960.

Fairbanks, G.: Systematic research in experimental phonetics: I. A theory of the speech mechanism as a servosystem. *J Speech Hear Disord, 19:*133-140, 1954.

Fernald, G.: *Remedial Techniques in Basic School Subjects.* New York, McGraw-Hill, 1939.

Filter, M. D.: Proprioceptive-tactile-kinesthetic feedback in voice therapy. *Language, Speech and Hearing Services in Schools,* American Speech and Hearing Association, *5:*149-151, 1974.

Fletcher, H.: *Speech and Hearing in Communication,* 2nd ed. New York, D. Van Nostrand, 1953, p. 86.

Flowers, Ann M.: Pioneers in speech pathology—Sara Stinchfield Hawk: Pioneer speech pathologist. *J Speech Hear Assoc Virginia, 8,* 1966.

Fucci, D. J., and Robertson, J. H.: "Functional" defective articulation: An oral sensory disturbance. *Perceptual and Motor Skills, 33:*711-714, 1971.

Gammon, Sylvia A., Smith, P., Daniloff, R. G., and Kim, C.: Articulation and stress/juncture production under oral anesthetization and masking. *J Speech Hear Res, 14:*271-282, 1971.

Gibson, J. J.: The mouth as an organ for laying hold on the environment. In Bosma, J. F. (Ed.): *Symposium on Oral Sensation and Perception.* Springfield, Thomas, 1967, pp. 111-136.

Gillingham, A., and Stillman, B.: *Remedial Training for Children with Specific Disability in Reading, Spelling, and Penmanship.* Cambridge, MA, Educators Publishing Service, 1960.

Gray, B. B., and England, G.: *Stuttering and the Conditioning Therapies.* Monterey, CA, The Monterey Institute for Speech and Hearing, 1969, p. iii.

Grossman, R. C., and Bosma, J. F.: Experimental oral sensory prosthesis. *J Dent Res, 42:*891, 1963.

Grossman, R. C., Hattis, B. F., and Ringel, R. L.: Oral tactile experience. *Arch Oral Biol, 10:*691-705, 1965.

Hahn, E. F.: A discussion of the moto-kinaesthetic method of speech correction. *Q J Speech, 25,* 1939.

Hahn, E. F.: The moto-kinaesthetic method of speech training. *J Except Children, 6,* 1940.

Hardy, J. C.: *Development of Neuromuscular Systems Underlying Speech Production. ASHA Report #5.* Washington, D. C.: American Speech and Hearing Association, 1970, pp. 49-68.

Hawk, Sara Stinchfield: Moto-kinaesthetic speech training for children. *J Speech Disord, 2,* 1937.

Hawk, Sara Stinchfield: Kinaesthetic factors in speech training. *Proceedings of the American Speech Correction Association.* Madison, Madison College Typing Co., 1938.

Hawk, Sara Stinchfield: The pre-school child with delayed or defective speech. *Pi Lambda Theta Journal,* 1939.

Hawk, Sara Stinchfield: Can a child be taught to talk? *J Speech Disord,* February, 1939.

Hawk, Sara Stinchfield: Moto-kinaesthetic training for children with speech handicaps. *J Except Children, 8,* 1941.

Hawk, Sara Stinchfield: Moto-kinaesthetic training for children with speech handicaps. *J Speech Disord, 7,* 1942.

Hawk, Sara Stinchfield: Moto-kinaesthetic speech training applied to visually handicapped children. *Outlook for the Blind, 38,* 1944.

Hawk, Sara Stinchfield: Speech training in a nursery school for visually handicapped children. *Outlook for the Blind, 39,* 1944.

Hawk, Sara Stinchfield: Genesis. The voice. *J Cal Speech and Hear Assoc 13,* 1964.

Heider, F. K., and Heider, G. M.: An experimental investigation of lipreading. *Psychol Monogr, 52:*124-153, 1940.

Henneman, E.: Organizaton of the motor system—a preview. In Mountcastle, V. B. (Ed.): *Med Physiol,* 12th ed. St. Louis, Mosby, 1968, Vol. II.

Hosokawa, H.: Proprioceptive innervation of striated muscle in the territory of cranial nerves. *Tex Rep Biol Med, 19:*405-464, 1961.

Humphrey, Tryphena: Reflex activity in the oral and facial area of the human fetus. In Bosma, J. F. (Ed.): *Symposium on Oral Sensation and Perception.* Springfield, Thomas, 1970, pp. 195-233.

Hutchinson, J. M., and Putnam, Anne H. B.: Aerodynamic aspect of sensory deprived speech. *J Acoust Soc Am, 56:* 1612-1617, 1974.

Hutton, C. L.: Combining auditory and visual stimuli in aural rehabilitation. *Volta Rev, 61:*316-319, 1959.

Hutton, C. L.: Aural rehabilitation. In Griffith, J.: *Persons with Hearing Loss.* Springfield, Thomas, 1969, pp. 109-137.

Konigsmark, B. W.: *Neuroanatomy of Speech. ASHA Reports #5.* Washington, D. C., American Speech and Hearing Association, 1970, pp. 3-19.

Larson, M. H.: *A Study of Lingual Sensory Characteristics Accompanying "Functional" Disorders of Articulation.* Unpublished doctoral thesis, University of Denver, 1955.

Leanderson, R. (Ed.): *On the Functional Organization of Facial Muscles in Speech.* Stockholm, Sweden: Departments of Otolaryngology and Clinical Neurophysiology, Karolinska Sjukhuset, 1972.

Leanderson, R., and Persson, A.: The effect of trigeminal nerve block on the articulatory EMG activity of facial muscles. Reprinted from *Acta Otolaryng,* 1972, in Leanderson, R. (Ed.): *On the Functional Organization of Facial Muscles in Speech.* Stockholm, Sweden, Karolinska Sjukhuset, 1972.

Liberman, A. M.: Some results of research in speech perception. *J Acoust Soc Am, 29:*117-123, 1957.

Light, J., Silverman, S. I., and Garfinkel, L.: The use of an intraoral training aid in the speech rehabilitation of laryngectomy patients. *J Prosthet Dent, 35:*430-439, 1976.

Locke, J.: Oral perception and articulation learning. *Percept Mot Skills, 26:*1259-1264, 1968.

McCall, G. N.: The assessment of lingual tactile sensation and perception. *J Speech Hear Disord, 34:*151-156, 1969.

McCroskey, R. L.: The relative contribution of auditory and tactile cues to certain aspects of speech. *South Speech J, 24:*84-90, 1958.

McDonald, E. T.: *Articulation Testing and Treatment: A Sensory-Motor Approach.* Pittsburgh, Stanwix House, 1967.

McDonald, E. T., and Aungst, L. F.: Studies in oral sensorimotor function. In Bosma, J. F. (Ed.): *Symposium on Oral Sensation and Perception.* Springfield, Thomas, 1967, pp. 202-220.

Matthews, P. B. C.: Muscle spindles and their motor control. *Physiol Rev, 44:*219-287, 1964.

May, Annette A., and Hudgens, D. A.: *Application of Selected Proprioceptive Neuromuscular Facilitation Techniques in the Treatment of Dysarthria.* Mini Seminar, American Speech and Hearing Association Convention, Chicago, 1977.

Montessori, M.: *The Montessori Method.* New York, Frederick A. Stokes, 1912.

Morley, M. E., and Fox, J.: Disorders of articulation: Theory and therapy. *Br J Disord Commun, 4:*151-165, 1969.

Mountcastle, V. B.: Physiology of sensory receptors: Introduction to sensory processes. In Mountcastle, V. B. (Ed.): *Medical Physiology,* 12th ed. St. Louis, Mosby, 1968, Vol. II.

Mountcastle, V. B., and Darian-Smith, I.: Neural mechanisms in somesthesia. In Mountcastle, V. B. (Ed.): *Medical Physiology,* 12th ed. St. Louis, Mosby, 1968, Vol. II.

Mysak, E. A.: A servo model for speech therapy. *J Speech Hear Disord, 24:* 144-149, 1959.

Mysak, E. D.: *Speech Pathology and Feedback Theory.* Springfield, Thomas, 1966.

National Institute of Neurological Disease and Blindness: *A Decade of Progress,* 1961.

O'Neill, J. J.: Contributions of the visual components of oral symbols to speech comprehension. *J Speech Hear Disord, 19:*429-439, 1954.

Osgood, C. E.: A behavioristic analysis of perception and language as cognitive phenomena. In Buckley, W. F.: *Modern Systems Research for the Behavioral Scientist*. Chicago, Aldine, 1968.

Patton, Francis E.: A comparison of kinaesthetic sensibility of speech-defective and normal speaking children. *J Speech Disord, 7,* 1942.

Perkins, W. H.: *Speech Pathology, An Applied Behavioral Science.* St. Louis, Mosby, 1971, p. 30.

Press, Judith: *Oral Form Discrimination Ability of Children Misarticulating R and S.* Master's Thesis, University of California, Sacramento, 1975.

Poole, Irene: Genetic development of articulation of consonant sounds in speech. *Elementary English Rev, 11:*159-161, 1934.

Pfoff, P. L.: The moto-kinaesthetic method applied to aphasics. *J Speech Disord, 5,* 1940.

Putnam, Anne H. B., and Ringel, R. L.: Tongue and lip sensation in relation to a trigeminal nerve block. *Purdue University Contributed Papers #2,* 1973, pp. 1-5.

Putnam, Anne H. B., and Ringel, R. L.: A cineradiographic study of articulation in two talkers with temporarily-induced oral sensory deprivation. *J Speech Hear Res, 19:*247-266, 1976.

Remblisz, Linda S., and Gribin, Sabra, A.: *Neuromuscular Facilitation Therapeutic Techniques in Treating the Dysarthric Patient.* Mini seminar, New Jersey Speech and Hearing Association, 1977 (Mimeographed copy available from authors, Children's Specialized Hospital, Westfield, N. J.).

Ringel, R. L., and Steer, M. D.: Some effects of tactile and auditory alterations on speech output. *J Speech Hear Res, 6:*369-378, 1963.

Ringel, R. L., and Ewanowski, S. J.: Oral perception: I. Two-point discrimination. *J Speech Hear Res, 8:*389-398, 1965.

Ringel, R. L., Burk, K. W., and Scott, Cheryl, M.: Tactile perception: Form discrimination in the mouth. *Br J Disord Commun, 3:*150-155, 1968.

Ringel, R. L.: *Oral Sensation and Perception: A Selective Review. ASHA Reports #5.* Washington, D. C., American Speech and Hearing Association, 1970, pp. 188-206.

Ringel, R. L., Putnam, Anne H. B., and Williams, W.: *Oral Sensory Perception.* Short Course Presented at the California Speech and Hearing Association Conference, 1974.

Rootes, T. P., and MacNeilage, P. F.: Some speech perception and production tests of a patient with impairment of somesthetic perception and motor function. In Bosma, J. F. (Ed.): *Symposium on Oral Sensation and Perception.* Springfield, Thomas, 1967, pp. 310-317.

Ruscello, D. M., and Lass, N. J.: *Articulation improvement and oral tactile changes in children.* Unpublished manuscript, West Virginia University, 1972.

Rutherford, D., and McCall, G.: Testing oral sensation and perception in persons with dysarthria. In Bosma, J. F. (Ed.): *Symposium in Oral*

Sensation and Perception. Springfield, Thomas, 1967, pp. 188-201.

Ryan, T. A.: Interrelations of the sensory systems in perception. *Psychol Bull, 37*:659-698, 1940.

Samuelson, E. E. (Ed.): *New Aids and Materials for Teaching Lip-Reading.* Washington, D. C., American Society for the Hard of Hearing, 1943.

Schilder, P.: *The Image and Appearance of the Human Body.* New York, Intl Univs Pr, 1950.

Scott, Cheryl M., and Ringel, R. L.: Articulation without oral sensory control. *J Speech Hear Res, 14*:804-818, 1971.

Shelton, R. L., Arndt, W. B., and Hetherington, J. J.: Testing oral stereognosis. In Bosma, J. F. (Ed.): *Symposium on Oral Sensation and Perception.* Springfield, Thomas, 1967, pp. 221-243.

Sim, J. M.: *Speech Accommodation to Artificial Changes in Volume of the Palate in Normal Children.* Master's Thesis, U of Washington Pr, 1966.

Sommers, R. K., and Kane, Ann R.: Functional articulation disorders. In Dickson, S. (Ed.): *Communication Disorders: Remedial Principles and Practices.* Glenview, IL, Scott F, 1974.

Speech Foundation of America. *On Stuttering, Its Treatment.* Memphis, Speech Foundation of America, 1960, pp. 27-28.

Stinchfield, Sara: Binaural hearing and delayed speech development. *Harvard Teachers Record, 5,* 1935.

Stinchfield, Sara, and Young, Edna Hill: *Children With Delayed or Defective Speech: Moto-Kinesthetic Factors in Their Training.* Stanford, U Pr, 1938.

Strauss, A. A., and Lehtinen, L. W.: *Psychopathology and Education of the Brain-Injured Child.* New York, Grune & Stratton, 1947.

Telage, K., and Fucci, D.: Vibrotactile stimulation: A future clinical tool for speech pathologists. *J Speech and Hear Disord, 38*:442-447, 1973.

Templin, Mildred C.: *Certain Language Skills in Children.* Minneapolis: U of Minn Pr, 1957.

Thorndike-Barnhardt Comprehensive Desk Dictionary. New York, Doubleday, 1951.

Tjomsland, Lily M.: *Feel It and Say It.* New Richmond, WI, Whitehaven, 1968.

Tobias, J. V.: Relative occurrence of phonemes in American English. *J Acoust Soc Am, 31*:631, 1959.

Travis, L. E.: The pedagogical significance of the moto-kinaesthetic method. *J Speech Hear Disord, 15,* 1940.

Tyson, J. D.: *The Role of the Parietal Lobe in Speech.* Unpublished doctoral dissertation, University of Denver, 1954.

Van Riper, C., and Irwin, J. V.: *Voice and Articulation.* Englewood Cliffs, P-H, 1958.

Van Riper, C.: Behavior and modification: An overview. In *Conditioning in Stuttering Therapy.* Memphis, Speech Foundation of America, 1970, p. 9.

Vaughn, Gwenyth R.: *Moto-Kinesthetic Stimulations.* Unpublished doctoral dissertation, Universidad Nacional Autonoma de Mexico, 1951.

Wapner, S., and Werner, H. (Eds.): *The Body Percept.* New York, Random, 1965.

Webster's Seventh New Collegiate Dictionary. Springfield, MA, Merriam, 1965, p. 15a.

Wellman, Beth L., Case, Ida M., Mengert, Ida G., and Bradbury, Dorothy E.: Speech sounds of young children. *University of Iowa Studies in Child Welfare, 5,* 1936.

Wilentz, Joan S.: *The Senses of Man.* New York, Thomas Y. Crowell, 1968.

Wilhelm, C. C.: *The Effects of Oral Form Recognition Training on Articulation in Children.* Unpublished doctoral dissertation, University of Kansas, 1966. In Ruscello, D. M., and Lass, N. N.: *Articulation Improvement and Oral Tactile Changes in Children.* Unpublished manuscript, West Virginia University, 1972.

Williams, W. N., and LaPointe, L. L.: Correlations between oral form recognition and lingual touch sensitivity. *Percept Mot Skills, 32:*840-842, 1971a.

Williams, W. N., and LaPointe, L. L.: Intra-oral recognition of geometric forms by normal subjects. *Percept Mot Skills, 32:*419-426, 1971b.

Woodward, M. F.: Linguistic Methodology in Lip Reading. *John Tracy Clinic Research Paper, #IV.* Los Angeles, John Tracy Clinic, 1957.

Wylie, Ruth C.: *The Self Concept: A Critical Survey of Pertinent Research Literature.* Lincoln, U of Neb Pr, 1961.

Yale, Caroline A.: *Formation and Development of Elementary English Sounds.* Northampton, MA, Clarke School for the Deaf, 1946.

Young, Edna Hill: The moto-kinaesthetic method of speech training. *J Speech Disord, 5,* 1940.

Young, Edna Hill: Better help for speech beginnings. *Am J Dis Child, 68,* 1944.

Young, Edna Hill: The beginnings of speech. *Western Speech, 9,* 1945.

Young, Edna Hill, Van Tine, R., Shutts, R. E., Woellhof, R., and Winchester, R.: *The Moto-Kinesthetic Method.* (The film, made in 1951, has been lost. The quotation was taken from Mrs. Young's notes which go with this film.)

Young, Edna Hill: A personal experience with speech. *J Speech Hear Disord, 23,* 1958.

Young, Edna Hill: The moto-kinesthetic approach to the prevention of speech defects, including stuttering. *J Speech Hear Disord, 30,* 1965.

Young, Edna Hill: Values of early speech training. *The Voice. J Cal Speech Hear Assoc, 16,* 1967.

Young, Edna Hill, and Hawk, Sara Stinchfield: *Moto-Kinesthetic Speech Training.* Stanford, Stanford U Pr, 1955, p. 11.

Zaliouk, A.: A visual-tactile system of phonetic symbolization. *J Speech Hear Disord, 19,* 1954.

Zlatin, Marsha A.: Development of speech, language, auditory and oral function in the presence of congenital sensory neuropathy. In Bosma, J. B. (Ed.): *Third Symposium on Oral Sensation and Perception.* Springfield, Thomas, 1972, pp. 381-390.

INDEX

G

H

P

R

S